HYPOTHERMIA

HYPOTHERMIA
Death By Exposure

William W. Forgey M.D.

ICS BOOKS, INC.
MERRILLVILLE, INDIANA

616.9
F763h

HYPOTHERMIA

Copyright © 1985 by William W. Forgey, M.D.

85-0606

10 9 8 7 6 5 4 3 2 1

Printed in U.S.A.

Published by:
ICS Books, Inc.
1000 E. 80th Place
Merrillville, IN 46410

Distributed by:
Stackpole Books
Cameron and Kelker Street
Harrisburg, PA 17105

Library of Congress Cataloging in Publication Data

Forgey, William W.,
    Hypothermia : death by exposure.

    Bibliography: p.
    Includes index.
    1. Hypothermia.   I. Title   [DNLM: 1. Hypothermia.
WD 670 F721h]
RC88.5.F67 1984   616.9'89   84-19803
ISBN 0-934802-10-6

DEDICATION

This book is dedicated to my good friend and colleague Paul Petzoldt, for his life-long service to outdoor education. A noted mountaineer, he became the first Outward Bound instructor in the United States, was the founder of NOLS (The National Outdoor Leadership School), and is currently a founding member and trustee of the Wilderness Education Association.

The Wilderness Education Association, which provides a curriculum for outdoor leadership training and certification at participating universities and colleges across the United States, embodies the dedication which Mr. Petzoldt has demonstrated to our current outdoor leaders and through them to future generations for safe and ecologically sound wilderness travels.

Naturam expella furca licet tamen usque recurrit*

Although nature and natural causes be forced and resisted ever so much, yet at last they will have their own way again.

George Best
The Third Frobisher Voyage 1578

Table of Contents

PREFACE

The preparation of this book required 5 years of research, including participation and attendance of many seminars, searching the medical and popular outdoor literature, and personal conversations with many authorities on the subject of hypothermia and the cold related injuries. Over 200 references to the subject have been synthesized into this book. Many discrepancies in both the scientific and popular outdoor literature had to be studied and decisions made with regard to nearly every aspect of the material contained herein. The study of hypothermia has many controversial aspects. Many bits of information are at divergence from study to study.

Some authorities become impressed with a particular aspect of this subject and over-react to certain methods of prevention and treatment that may not be practical under field conditions. And, at times there is probably no best solution to a field hypothermia emergency. I have carefully chosen the most logical approaches to all aspects of this subject based upon my technical research and my personal experience from many trips to the Canadian sub-arctic during the winter months. I have attempted to present a balanced view of the controversial aspects of this subject.

My closest calls to hypothermia have never come on these Arctic journeys. But well I remember a particular caving trip in Southern Indiana, a canoe trip in North Carolina and another in Upper State New York, and a winter hike on Grandfather Mountain in North Carolina -- events that occurred over the past 25 years that gave me a healthy respect for the cold, for freezing weather and wet clothes, for sudden swims in icy water.

The treatment of hypothermia has been a particular interest of mine, probably because of my interest in various aspects of caring for those engaged in wilderness travel. I hope that my approaches to the field management of these injuries will be of help to my fellow outdoors travelers.

vi   Death By Exposure

ACKNOWLEDGEMENTS

If it were not for many others, this book could not have been written. Directly influencing me were two great outdoorsmen and writers, the late Calvin Rutstrum and the late Sigurd F. Olson.

My first trip into the barrens of Arctic Canada during the winter was made feasible through the writings of Calvin Rutstrum's book *Paradise Below Zero*. Rutstrum had two great attributes as a writer. He only wrote what he knew about and he was a man of great outdoor skills.

The writings of Sigurd F. Olson are inspirational to anyone who loves the northwoods and beyond. His personal help in assisting me organize my earliest trips into the winter Arctic made possible my many encounters with that wonderful country. Of particular note were the efforts In our behalf by his friend Major General Elliott Roger, Canadian Armed Forces (Retired), which ranged from special permits to meeting our planes and trains and purchasing supplies.

Robert and Judy Pilgrim Stewart of Winnipeg, Manitoba, have directly aided in the research for this book and in bunking down our many crew members in their home during our staging periods before leaving for the north country. Their son Paget and daughters Jennie and Victoria have played host to over 50 of us during the past 12 years.

There are many great physicians and scientific researchers who have added immense knowledge to the field of hypothermia. I have been particularly impressed by the writings of Marlin Kreider, M.D., William Mills, M.D., Cameron Bangs, M.D., Murray Hamlet, D.V.M., Robert Pozos, Ph.D., James Lipton, Ph.D., Loren Johnson, M.D., Bradford Washburn, Ph.D., the late Theodore Lathrop, M.D., and the late Robert Bullard, Ph.D. The fact that the latter two men lost their lives while in the field is indicative of the fact that the most knowledgeable persons can meet with insurmountable disaster -- something we must all respect.

And finally, I must pay particular attention to those who have travelled north with me during the winter -- frequently so I could try some new technique or engage them in pulling supplies under some rather awesome circumstances. This has frequently taken courage and certainly trust in my judgement -- which has often been based upon those mentioned in the paragraphs above. Notably I wish to thank Steve McClain for that first trip, Jeff St. Claire for help on a bitter cold trip with many heavy loads, Ralph Ehresman for his 5 trips, and Greg Filter, James Ross, Scott McDonald, and Roy Becker -- who have logged over 7 months field time each, and Joe Sanders for tolerating my vapor barrier experiments.

A particular thanks to Joe Kowal of the Polar Hotel in Churchill, Manitoba, for many years of assistance in storing our supplies, feeding us, hauling us around, and in preparing for our departures and returns from the bush.

A personal thanks to Tom Todd, my publisher and editor, who has accompanied me on many trips to the bush. Few authors have been blessed with such assistance.

William W. Forgey, M.D.
Merrillville, Indiana
July 1984

1. HYPOTHERMIA

Hypothermia has become well established as a major cause of deaths that occur amongst outdoor travelers. Its significance for all of us has been emphasized by Dr. Richard W. Besdine of the Harvard Medical School, who has stated that 2.5 million Americans are at risk of dying from hypothermia each year. This number is large due to the many causes of low body temperature beyond those encountered by the sportsman. Elderly people whose apartment heat has been reduced are most vulnerable. Unfortunately, many people make trips in their car dressed to arrive, not to survive roadside emergencies. Falling into cold water results in a rapid loss of body heat. Some illnesses and many medications can predispose people to hypothermia. Alcohol and abused drugs contribute to cold weather deaths.

While this is a problem of universal importance, this book has been designed for the outdoor traveler -- and, if necessary, the rescuer. For outdoorspersons, hypothermia is the most potentially important wilderness danger which they are likely to encounter. Hypothermic sports victims tend to be young, have suffered an accident or become lost, or to have been unprepared for the weather conditions which befell them.

The term "hypothermia" has replaced the expression "exposure" in both the popular and medical literature. The former describes what is termed a pathological condition -- it is an illness, in this case an illness caused by the body's core (or inner) temperature being lowered below normal to the point that the person is ill. The term "exposure" refers to the method by which the person becomes hypothermic.

A person can be classified as hypothermic when their core temperature is below 95°F (35°C). Hypothermia is classified by rapidity of onset and by the resulting degree of core temperature drop. These classifications are useful for choosing a therapeutic approach and for establishing a prognosis.

There are several aspects of the problem that must be understood. First are the physical forces in the environment that may cause loss of body heat. Second, the methods of heat production and protection that the body has at its disposal. Third, studying the physiology of hypothermia to understand the pathology that occurs when a victim becomes hypothermic. Fourth, ways of assisting the body in preserving or adding to its heat source. Fifth, developing methods of diagnosing and treating the hypothermia victim in the field with a look to what will have to happen during subsequent hospital care if the victim is to survive. And sixth, understanding the other cold related injuries that can occur and how they should be treated.

2. ENVIRONMENTAL INFLUENCES

The Physical Laws of Nature

The physical laws of nature can be bent to our commands, but they can never be ignored. This is particularly true when it comes to man's survival in the environment. A warm-blooded mammal such as man is scientifically termed a "homeotherm." This is an organism that must maintain its body temperature within a narrow range (101° to 96°F or 38° to 35.5°C) to properly function. The organism internally generates heat to accomplish this. The environment can both aid and hinder by adding more heat (either too little or too much), or by sapping heat away.

It is within this range that the body enzyme systems work the most efficiently. A wider range can be tolerated, but decreased efficiency of the vital processes in the body result. At the extreme ends of the tolerable range, death results from the inactivation and destruction of the inter-connected enzymatic functions.

Figure 1 indicates the physiological responses at various core temperature levels and also shows typical behavioral activity that might provide a clue to core temperature. It should be emphasized that the field diagnosis of hypothermia can be very difficult. Most experts will stress that one cannot rely on these indicated symptoms. Dr. Cameron Bangs, a noted mountain rescue and hypothermia expert, relates a story about a victim being pulled from a crevasse who could walk, talk intelligently, yet only to collapse with a measured core temperature of 77°F (25°C)!

An environmental or ambient temperature of lower than 77°F (25°C) results in a lowering of the core temperature of a naked human, unless either a mental or physiological response to counter that drop occurs.

The behavioral aspects of preventing core temperature drop is the essence of outdoor survival technique. Indeed, it can be complex. There are many ideas on proper insulation, new development of materials, and basically divergent concepts such as "breathabil-

SIGNS AND SYMPTOMS OF HYPOTHERMIA

CORE TEMP.	SIGNS AND SYMPTOMS
99° to 97°F (37° to 36°C)	Normal temperature range Shivering may begin
97° to 95°F (36° to 35°C)	Cold sensation, goose bumps, unable to perform complex tasks with hands, shivering can be mild to severe, skin numb
95° to 93°F (35° to 34°C)	Shivering intense, muscle incoordination becomes apparent, movements slow and labored, stumbling pace, mild confusion, may appear alert, unable to walk 30 ft. line properly — BEST FIELD TEST FOR EARLY HYPOTHERMIA
93° to 90°F (34° to 32°C)	Violent shivering persists, difficulty speaking, sluggish thinking, amnesia starts to appear and may be retrograde, gross muscle movements sluggish, unable to use hands, stumbles frequently, difficulty speaking, signs of depression
90° to 86°F 32° to 30°C)	Shivering stops in chronic hypothermia, exposed skin blue or puffy, muscle coordination very poor with inability to walk, confusion, incoherent, irrational behavior, BUT MAY BE ABLE TO MAINTAIN POSTURE AND THE APPEARANCE OF PSYCHOLOGICAL CONTACT
86° to 82°F (30° to 27.7°C)	Muscles severely rigid, semiconscious, stupor, loss of psychological contact, pulse and respirations slow, pupils can dilate
82° to 78°F (27 to 25.5°C)	Unconsciousness, heart beat and respiration erratic, pulse and heart beat may be inapparent, muscle tendon reflexes cease
78° to 75°F (25° to 24°C)	Pulmonary edema, failure of cardiac and respiratory centers, probable death, DEATH MAY OCCUR BEFORE THIS LEVEL
64°F (17.7°C)	Lowest recorded temperature of chronic hypothermia survivor, Chicago 1951
48.2°F (9°C)	Lowest recorded temperature of induced hypothermia in surgical patient with survival, 1958

FIGURE 1   "SIGNS AND SYMPTOMS OF HYPOTHERMIA"

ity'' and ''vapor barrier'' that we may wish to study from a physiological viewpoint. But there can be little doubt that the behavioral aspect of protecting our thin skins from the diversity of environments surrounding us is the most important aspect of enabling us to survive in any but a tropic environment. The migration of man from his point of origin necessitated his advance mentally to the level where tools and clothing could be made. Once our nakedness was covered, we could start to explore our globe and hope to survive the environments which we would encounter.

The environmental methods of heat transfer basically include radiation, conduction, evaporation, and convection. Variations of these basic physical events are: loss through the physiology of respiration and the bellows effect of clothing and sleeping bags.

Radiation

Heat is discharged directly from the body by the emission of infrared energy. Actually, radiation heats a surrounding micro-environment that convection can then strip away from the body. Radiation can also add heat to the body, directly from the sun, or through reflection, even from snow fields, and from other sources of radiant energy. Fires can provide radiant warmth as well as convection heat -- i.e. hot air.

Areas of potential radiation loss will be those areas that are: (1) exposed to the environment, (2) have large blood supplies, (3) are unable to restrict or minimize local blood supply significantly to prevent radiant heat loss. Radiant loss can occur from any un-covered body surface, but the head is the most obvious location for radiant heat loss. The uncovered head can lose up to one-half of the body's total heat production at 39°F (4°C).

Protection from radiation loss can be accomplished by reflec-tive materials, or any occlusive covering. For emergency use several products have been developed. Plastic sheeting with a fine film of aluminum was developed in the mid-1960's to reflect infrared radi-ation loss. See discussion of this and other radiation protection fabrics in the section on metallized plastic sheets on page 102.

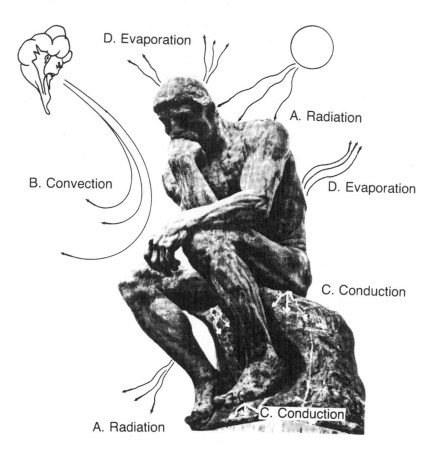

FIGURE 2   "MECHANISMS OF HEAT TRANSFER WITH THE ENVIRONMENT"
The mechanisms of heat transfer between man and the environment include: A. *Radiation* - heat transferred by electromagnetic waves from warm to cooler objects; B. *Convection* - heat transfer by molecules of air or fluid moving between areas of unequal temperature; C. *Conduction* - heat exchange between objects in contact; D. *Evaporation* - heat loss by water molecules diffusing from the body surface, by sweating, and by environmental wetting when this water changes from a liquid to a vapor state. The above methods are further explained in the text.

Conduction

Conduction is the direct transfer of heat from one object to another. Conductive heat loss from a human is most often the direct transfer of heat from the body to a cold surface, such as snow, cold ground, or water. Reduction of conductive heat loss is through insulation.

Insulation is generally a form of trapped air space. A large air space will allow heat drain by convection, so that the air space to be an effective insulator must be divided into multiple and small cells. For example, sleeping on an air mattress on the cold ground provides only slight insulation, while the same thickness of a foam pad can provide considerable protection. The concept of insulation is not that simple and we must return to it in greater depth, but let us acknowledge that conduction loss will be minimized by insulation of some sort. The degree of heat loss due to conduction will depend upon the surface area of the individual exposed to the "cold surface", the quality of the insulation between the two, and the temperature of both the individual and the cold surface.

The most profound conduction loss can potentially occur when submerged in cold water. An immersed individual in still water will lose heat by conduction at a rate 20 times faster than a dry individual in still air at the same temperature. This loss is so profound that it can cause the rapid development of hypothermia in a victim immersed in water colder than 68°F (20°C) -- a condition termed "acute hypothermia." This differs from the "chronic hypothermia" which outdoor travelers can develop from other than immersion situations. Generally, acute hypothermia develops in less than 6 hours, frequently less than 2 hours. The term "acute hypothermia" is regarded as synonymous with "immersion hypothermia."

Many insulating materials lose their protective properties when wet. Wool is one of the best insulating materials available, yet when it absorbs one-third of its weight it loses much of its insulation capability. Cotton is a very poor insulator even when merely damp.

Its use in the outdoors, even in denim jeans, should therefore be avoided. The use of cotton clothing can and does lead to survival tragedies due to its poor insulating ability. The section on clothing deals with many new fabrics which can prevent conduction heat loss, even when damp.

Conduction can be an insidious method of heat loss. Many people have heard that snow is a good insulator. But this insulation is at or below 32 degrees Fahrenheit. If the local temperature has been minus 20 degrees for several days, then the snow is minus 20 degrees in that area. Plunging along with inadequate foot insulation in snow of that temperature can lead to disaster.

Increasing the surface of contact with the ground, such as sitting or laying down, means more heat will be lost than if a small area of contact, such as the foot, is involved. Many types of clothing have insulation that can be crushed when lying on it. If this were to happen, the trapped air space is decreased and the insulation ability of the material is compromised. When resting on the ground, treat that cold ground as an enemy and expect that your clothing will frequently be inadequate protection when crushed against it. In an emergency, full use of "relatively" better insulation than surface rocks, packed earth or snow must be attempted with use of insulated pads, sleeping bags, extra clothing, packs, branches, leaves and grass, or even loose dirt beneath the victim. This should provide as much protection as possible against a continuous heat loss by conduction from the victim to the ground.

Evaporation

When water changes from a liquid to a gas it must absorb heat called the "latent heat of vaporization" or "latent heat of evaporation" to accomplish this change in its physical state. There is no change in the temperature of the substance, but there is an energy requirement to make this change from the liquid to gaseous state. This results in a consumption or loss of heat. While this is a valuable method of lowering body core temperature during times of high heat stress, it can become a liability during cold weather. The latent heat of vaporization is .54 kcal per gram of water, or 245 kcal per pound. This represents a considerable loss of heat and significant energy consumption if that heat must be replaced.

While sweating is a primary method of the body to reduce heat loss through the principle of latent heat of vaporization, this same principle may cost the body precious heat when wet clothes are drying on the victim, or moisture is drying from exposed skin surfaces. The production of sweat, or the accidental wetting of clothing from the environment, can thus reduce the effectiveness of insulation in two ways. One is through heat consumed by water during the evaporation process. The other is adding to heat loss through increased conduction through wet, less effective insulation. Rescue methods have attempted to prevent unnecessary loss of heat during the evaporation process. A method strongly advocated is to place the wet victim in a plastic (or otherwise water impermeable barrier) to prevent evaporation. *This will work only if outside additional insulation is provided, because the continued massive heat loss from conduction could soon prove fatal, regardless of the heat loss saved by blocking the latent heat of vaporization consumption.*

Latent heat of vaporization is entirely separate from heat required to thaw frozen water. This is called the latent heat of crystallization, but it plays virtually no significant role, even in the rescue of a victim with frozen clothing. In fact, frozen sleeping bags, or a shell of frozen clothing on a recent immersion victim in subfreezing weather, can aid the survival process by producing a wind proof barrier from the environment. The latent heat of crystallization IS a significant figure when dealing with the eating of snow. This subject is discussed further on page 30.

Convection

Both water and air are generally not still and in this another mechanism of heat loss can occur, loss by convection. The body is constantly warming a thin layer of water or air next to it, thus

FAHRENHEIT WIND CHILL EQUIVALENT TEMPERATURE

TEMPERATURE FAHRENHEIT

Wind Speed MPH	50	40	35	30	25	20	15	10	5	0	-5	-10	-15	-20	-25	-30	-35	-40	-45	-50	-55	-60
Calm	50	40	35	30	25	20	15	10	5	0	-5	-10	-15	-20	-25	-30	-35	-40	-45	-50	-55	-60
5	48	37	33	27	21	16	12	6	1	-5	-11	-15	-20	-26	-31	-36	-41	-47	-52	-57	-65	-70
10	40	28	21	16	9	4	-2	-9	-15	-24	-27	-33	-38	-46	-52	-58	-64	-70	-75	-83	-90	-95
15	36	22	16	9	1	-5	-11	-18	-25	-32	-40	-45	-51	-58	-65	-72	-77	-85	-90	-99	-105	-110
20	32	18	12	4	-4	-10	-17	-25	-32	-39	-46	-53	-60	-67	-75	-82	-89	-96	-102	-110	-115	-120
25	30	16	7	0	-7	-15	-22	-29	-37	-44	-52	-59	-67	-74	-83	-88	-96	-104	-111	-118	-125	-135
30	28	13	5	-2	-11	-18	-26	-33	-41	-48	-56	-63	-70	-79	-87	-94	-101	-109	-115	-125	-130	-140
35	27	11	3	-4	-13	-20	-27	-35	-43	-51	-60	-67	-72	-82	-90	-98	-105	-113	-120	-129	-135	-146
40	26	10	1	-6	-15	-21	-29	-37	-45	-53	-62	-69	-76	-85	-94	-100	-107	-115	-125	-132	-140	-150

Exposed Flesh Can Freeze in 60 Seconds

Exposed Flesh Can Freeze in 30 Seconds

FIGURE 3A   "WIND CHILL CHART - FAHRENHEIT"

NOTE 1.   The above chart has been based upon the Siple Equation and reflects Wind Chill Equivalent temperatures in Fahrenheit.

NOTE 2.   At low wind speeds, relative humidity and radiant heat are more important than wind speed in determining equivalent temperature comfort.

NOTE 3.   Most charts indicate that at wind speeds over 40 mph there is little additional wind chill effect. This is a reflection of an error in the basic equation at these higher wind speeds and is not correct. Heat loss IS magnified by these higher wind speeds, but the chart is an accurate indicator of equivalent temperature at speeds lower than 40 mph.

WIND CHILL (EQUIVALENT) TEMPERATURE

WIND SPEED — KILOMETERS PER HOUR	OUTDOOR AIR TEMPERATURE — DEGREES CELSIUS																
	20	16	12	8	4	0	-4	-8	-12	-16	-20	-24	-28	-32	-36	-40	-44
6	20	16	12	8	4	0	-4	-8	-12	-16	-20	-24	-28	-32	-36	-40	-44
10	18	14	9	5	0	-4	-8	-13	-17	-22	-26	-31	-35	-40	-44	-49	-53
20	16	11	5	0	-5	-10	-15	-21	-26	-31	-36	-42	-47	-50	-57	-63	-68
30	14	9	3	-3	-8	-14	-20	-25	-31	-37	-43	-48	-54	-60	-65	-71	-77
40	13	7	1	-5	-11	-17	-23	-29	-35	-41	-47	-53	-59	-65	-71	-77	-83
50	13	7	0	-6	-12	-18	-25	-31	-37	-43	-49	-56	-62	-68	-74	-80	-87
60	12	6	0	-7	-13	-19	-26	-32	-39	-45	-51	-58	-64	-70	-77	-83	-89

FIGURE 3B   "WIND CHILL CHART - CELSIUS"

NOTE 1.   The above chart has been based upon the Siple Equation and reflects Wind Chill Equivalent temperatures in Celsius degrees. Wind speed is kilometers per hour.

See also notes 2 and 3 under the Fahrenheit Wind Chill Chart on page 10.

forming a micro-environment with a higher temperature that surrounds it and protects it from the lower ambient temperature of the
environment. The slightest disturbance of this thin layer of warmth
strips it away by convection. Thus, this warm layer of air or water
is removed easily by wind, current, or by body movement and this
heat is lost. This micro-layer must then be reheated. A continuous
stripping action of the micro-environment will cause a continuous
loss of heat from the body.

The importance of wind or water movement is hard to em-
phasize adequately. At very cold ambient temperatures considerable
heat loss will result to warm the micro-environment. Movement of
this air mass greatly accelerates this loss and, hence, the importance
of the wind-chill table demonstrating a relative temperature level.
This type of table can put the danger of the cold/wind combination
into terms that are commonly understood, namely degrees above
or below zero Fahrenheit.

This expression of "wind chill factor" has been a great aid
in warning people of the dangers of convection coupled with cold
ambient temperature. It is based upon work performed by C. F.
Passel and P. A. Siple in the Antarctic during the winter of 1941.
In their experiment the time was measured to freeze cylinders of
water under different cold weather conditions. They developed a
formula that expressed heat loss as a function of wind speed and
air temperature. As mentioned above, in the United States this
expresssion is given in degrees above or below zero Fahrenheit.
Figure 3A demonstrates a wind chill factor chart using these terms
and illustrates the danger to exposed flesh at various wind chill
temperatures.

U.S. wind chill charts have been developed from mathematical
application of the National Weather Service formula (Technical
Procedures Bulletin No. 165, June 15, 1976), commonly called the
Siple equation. This equation has an error in that wind speeds at
very low level demonstrate an exaggerated heat loss, while wind
speeds above 45 miles per hour may cause little additional effect.
This is not true, but many wind chill charts which you will see will

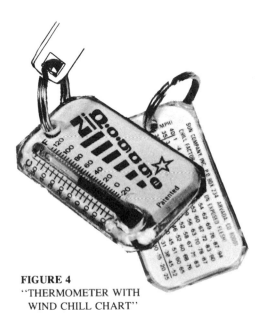

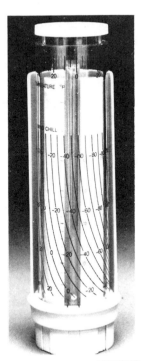

FIGURE 4
"THERMOMETER WITH
WIND CHILL CHART"

FIGURE 5
"TAYLOR WIND CHILL
INSTRUMENT"

indicate "Wind speeds above 40 mph have little additional effect."
With regard to both comfort and amount of heat loss, winds above
this speed DO cause increasing heat loss at a particular temperature,
but for practical purposes this well established method of depicting
the relative effect of wind speed on temperature has proven a valuable aid.

The wind chill factor used in the United States should be more
correctly termed an "equivalent chill temperature" or ECT. The
values obtained by this method are frequently beyond the experience
of many people, especially when figures like -70°F (-56°C) are

reached. The wind chill factor is actually a reflection of the rate of cooling due to convection heat loss. It is not an actual temperature. Some people assume incorrectly that objects can cool down to the wind chill equivalent temperature if left outside. This is not possible as an object will NOT cool to a lower temperature than its surroundings, i.e. the air temperature.

In Canada the temperature is measured in degrees Celsius and the wind speed in kilometers per hour. Throughout this book I have provided the English and the metric terms for ease in use by both U.S. and Canadian readers. Figure 3B is a wind chill equivalent chart designed for the metric system.

There are many easy to carry wind chill charts that have been reproduced on thermometers for easy calculation while in the field.

Taylor Instruments Company has developed a Wind Chill and Wind Speed Meter (see Figure 5) that is light weight (4.8 oz.), inexpensive ($21.95), and easily hand held. This self contained device measures wind speed and temperature, and has a mechanism whereby the user directly reads the wind chill equivalent temperature, from a rotating scale that matches temperature to wind speed.

In Canada, where the use of metric has supplanted the miles per hour for wind speed and the Celsius degree has replaced the Fahrenheit degree, a different expression of wind chill is used. This expression, "watts per square meter per hour" is an accurate expression of the actual energy loss due to the movement of air and the ambient temperature. The term seems foreign to the American ear, as I am sure it did to the Canadian ear when they first converted to the metric system. But like all systems, with use one readily identifies the perceived degree of coldness with the wind chill factor, whether it is expressed in "wind chill equivalent degrees Fahrenheit" or "watts per square meter per hour."

The advantage to the Canadian system is that the value actually expresses the amount of heat loss. This heat loss is in watts, a term which describes energy. The normal expression of metabolic energy is kilocalorie. We generally call kilocalories "calories." Through-

WIND CHILL COOLING RATES

(Watts per Square Metre)

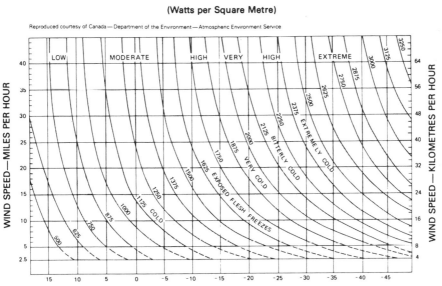

Reproduced courtesy of Canada—Department of the Environment—Atmospheric Environment Service

OUTDOOR AIR TEMPERATURE—DEGREES CELSIUS

Factor	Comments
700	Conditions considered comfortable when dressed for skiing.
1200	Conditions no longer pleasant for outdoor activities on overcast days.
1400	Conditions no longer pleasant for outdoor activities on sunny days.
1600	Freezing of exposed skin begins for most people depending on the degree of activity and the amount of sunshine.
2300	Conditions for outdoor travel such as walking become dangerous. Exposed areas of the face freeze in less than one minute for the average person.
2700	Exposed flesh will freeze within half a minute for the average person.

To determine the Wind Chill Factor follow the temperature across and the wind speed up until the two lines intersect. For example, at -10°C with a wind speed of 32 kilometers per hour, the point of intersection lies between 1500 and 1625, or approximately 1570.

It is not recommended that factors be calculated for wind speeds below 8 kilometers per hour since it is difficult to determine wind chill factors at these speeds because other factors, such as relative humidity, become important.

FIGURE 6   "WIND CHILL COOLING RATES GRAPH"

The actual wind chill cooling rates in watts per square meter per hour can be computed from the above graph. This figure can be converted into kcal of energy loss or wind chill comfort as indicated in the text.

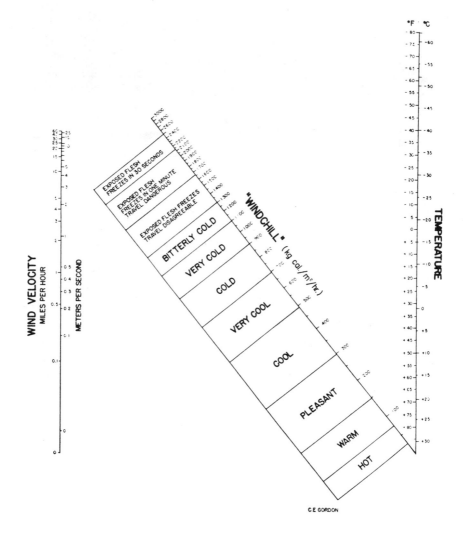

FIGURE 7   "WIND CHILL COOLING RATES NOMOGRAPH"

Another method of computing wind chill cooling rates in watts per square meter per hour is from the handy nomograph published by Consolazio, Johnson, and Marek in *"Metabolic Methods,"* C.V. Mosby Company, 1951, used by permission.

out the remainder of this book I will use the more correct expression kilocalories and abbreviate it "kcal." Watts can be converted to kcal by multiplying watts by .862. By entering the Canadian wind chill chart, it is possible to demonstrate the actual energy loss that can be converted to the number of kcal required to supply the amount of heat involved.

When using the Canadian wind chill chart several factors should be remembered. First, the table has been derived from the Siple equation, again showing some of the inaccuracies of very low wind speeds and of wind speeds above 45 mph (72 kilometers per hour). And second, the energy loss is computed per square meter of skin exposed. Of course, a square meter of skin would not be exposed during cold temperatures. The average adult male has 1.8 square meters of skin on his entire body. Only a small area of bare skin, namely parts of the head and occasionally the hands, would be expected to be exposed under very cold conditions.

At times nomograms are used in computing wind chill values. Reproduced as Figure 7 is a well known nomogram for calculating wind chill values in watts per square meter per hour. The boxes adjacent to the numerical readings provide a comfort index indicating coldness and exposed flesh freezing danger.

A major value in computing the wind chill factor is the determination of the degree of comfort and danger during exposure to the combined effects of temperature and wind speed. A general idea of the wind chill factor significance can be found by the following table:

FACTOR & COMMENTS
Watts per square meter per hour

700	Conditions considered comfortable when dressed for skiing.
1200	Conditions no longer pleasant for outdoor activities on overcast days.
1400	Conditions no longer pleasant for outdoor activities on sunny days.
1600	Freezing of exposed skin begins for most people depending on the degree of activity and the amount of sunshine.
2300	Conditions for outdoor travel such as walking become dangerous. Exposed areas of the face freeze in less than one minute for the average person.
2700	Exposed flesh will freeze within half a minute for the average person.

To accurately indicate degree of comfort, the ideal wind chill index would not only have to take into account ambient temperature and wind speed, but also the clothing worn, the activity level of the individual, and many other factors. The ideal wind chill index would take into account clothing distribution, insulation, body and skin temperature, metabolic heat production, heat loss from lungs, solar radiation, radiative heat loss, conductive heat loss, convective heat loss, while making assumptions for variations due to sex, age, state of health, and psychological attitude.

The immense amount of heat loss due to immersion in cold water is discussed in the sections on conduction and cold water immersion. Movement of water, or of the individual through water, also causes a convection heat loss. This has caused the development of special techniques for floating in cold water to minimize heat loss and increase survival chances (see section on Cold Water Immersion, pages 72-81).

3.   HEAT PRODUCTION

While heat is received from the environment in the form of radiation from the sun, and to a lesser degree from warm air convection and heated conduction sources, the main acquisition of heat comes from within. The basis of this heat is the food which we eat which provides the kcal of energy. These kcal are converted into various biochemical substrates that can be used to generate work and heat. The important bodily functions which produce heat can be considered under the topics of basal metabolic rate, nonshivering thermogenesis, specific dynamic action of food, volitional exercise, and the shivering response.

Basal Metabolic Rate, Nonshivering Thermogenesis, and the Specific Dynamic Action of Food

Heat is produced as a byproduct of the metabolism required by cells to survive. The amount of metabolic heat produced by various organ systems differs, as can be seen by Figure 8. This basal metabolic rate (BMR) differs by age, sex, and at times by race and exposure to cold or heat stress.

The various organ systems produce about 72% of the basal metabolic heat when at rest, but only contribute approximately 25% of total heat production during exercise. The BMR produces about 70 kcal/hour for the average weight (155 pound or 70 kilogram) man. Under conditions of cold stress the BMR can be increased by approximately 25%. This is probably effected by the release of a thyroid stimulating hormone, which increases the amount of the two active thyroid hormones in circulation, and by the increase in adrenal release of epinephrine and norepinephrine (adrenalin and noradrenalin).

The latter may cause increased utilization of "brown fat." It has been known that brown fat differs from normal fat or adipose tissue, which is a storage form of energy containing triglyceride and fatty acids. Brown fat is present in rodents and human infants; its presence in adults is now being studied. It appears to play a role

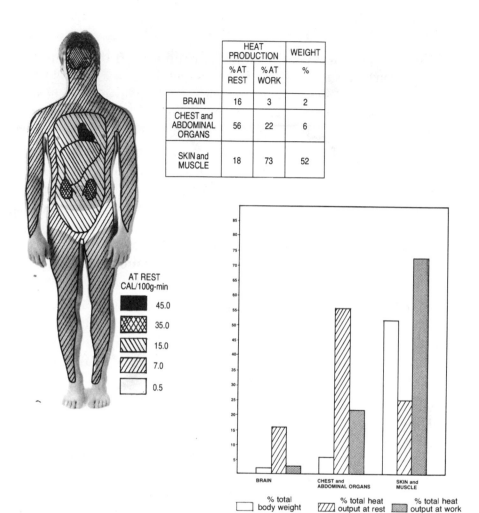

	HEAT PRODUCTION		WEIGHT
	% AT REST	% AT WORK	%
BRAIN	16	3	2
CHEST and ABDOMINAL ORGANS	56	22	6
SKIN and MUSCLE	18	73	52

AT REST
CAL/100g-min

■	45.0
▨	35.0
▧	15.0
▨	7.0
□	0.5

□ % total body weight   ▨ % total heat output at rest   ■ % total heat output at work

FIGURE 8   "PERCENT OF HEAT PRODUCTION VS. WEIGHT OF VARIOUS BODY TISSUES DURING WORK"

The above graph illustrates the percentage of body weight versus the amount of heat an organ system produces in the working individual. The brain composes 2% of body weight, produces 16% of body heat production when at rest, but this drops to 3% of total body heat in the working subject. The chest and abdominal organs are 6% of body weight, produce 56% of body heat at rest, but only 22% of total heat output in the working individual. Skin and muscle are 52% of the total body weight, produce 18% of heat output in a resting subject, but can produce 25% to 73% of heat production in a working person. Adopted from Auerbach and Geehr, *Management of Wilderness and Environmental Emergencies*, Macmillan, 1983, and Selkurt *Physiology 4th Ed*, 1976.

in generating heat -- heat produced by this means is termed "non-shivering thermogenesis." The total amount of heat produced in this fashion is minimal when compared to the amount of heat produced by volitional work and shivering, but it probably plays a role in the increased basal heat production noted during cold acclimatization.

The old saying, "we are what we eat" can be modified to "eat for heat." The source of metabolic and work generated heat is the energy locked in the carbohydrate, fat, and protein which we consume. It is these three nutrients that supply calories. It is important to obtain not only an adequate total number of calories per day based on expected requirements, but also a proper mix of these three nutrients should be consumed to derive the maximum benefit. This has a particular value with weight conscious backpackers who wish to obtain the most benefit for the least weight.

Nutritional Sources of Heat Production

CARBOHYDRATE

Carbohydrates consist of starches and sugars which are broken down into simple sugars called monosaccharides. The latter are absorbed from the intestines and transported directly to the liver by a closed circulatory system known as the portal system. The liver is responsible for maintaining a nearly constant supply of the monosaccharide "glucose" in the blood at all times. When glucose is absorbed after a meal or a candy tablet is ingested, the liver quickly converts it to glycogen. In turn, glycogen can be broken down into glucose during periods of fasting (which include any period during which no food is being digested). During rest, muscle tissue also forms glycogen, rather slowly, from the glucose liberated by the liver into the general systemic circulation, which is then stored in the muscle to be consumed during active periods.

As all carbohydrates are converted into glucose before being utilized by the body for energy, it makes no difference which of the various forms of carbohydrate are consumed. Starches take a little longer to digest and be absorbed in an experimental model in which the stomach is empty and glucose solution is compared to starch solution during uptake experiments. But in a human with food in the intestines, this starch will be broken down into sugars (monosaccharides) by the time the absorptive position in the intestines is reached -- and the speed of uptake will be virtually identical to pure glucose absorption.

One gram of carbohydrate produces 4 kcal of energy. This actually varies from 4.2 kcal per gram of starch to 3.7 kcal per gram of glucose, but the average used in dietetic computations is 4 kcal per gram of carbohydrate. The liver has a limited storage capacity for glycogen and when this excess is reached the adipose -- or fat forming tissue of the body -- does just what its name indicates: it forms fat. Usually 50% or more of the diet is supplied by carbohydrates. Carbohydrate intake is often the principle variable in weight loss or gain. A minimum of 5 grams (or 20 kcal) of carbohydrate per 100 kcal of total diet is required to prevent a condition known as ketosis (which results from the metabolism of fat components called "fatty acids" exclusively).

As mentioned above, the rapidity of uptake of sugar is not subject to tremendous changes in a human due to the type of sugar or starch, or even to the type of other fluid or food components with which it is consumed. There are many products on the market that claim they will replace blood sugar more rapidly than a regular sucrose tablet. This change in rapidity of uptake is minimal. In fact, the rapidity of uptake of sucrose over the more complex forms of carbohydrate, the starches, is virtually insignificant.

So, in other words, there is no super quick way to get sugar into the blood stream by mouth that does a much better job than a candy tablet.

The next shocker for many people is that once this sugar is in the blood stream, IT IS NOT AVAILABLE FOR INSTANT ENERGY. Many athletes, hikers, runners, and others will remark on how a candy bar provided them a quick energy pick up and that an "emergency energy lift" can and should be provided by carrying candy tablets or bars while hiking, etc. It has been known experimentally for a long time that this was not so. In the spring of 1982 the *New England Journal of Medicine* again published a research report that demonstrated that the energy level in a person was not linked to their blood sugar level. While it was known that long distance runners can have a low blood sugar, this low sugar level did not correlate with the work out-put, or even the feeling of fatigue. Replacing this sugar level to high normal did not further their ability to produce more work and it did not make them feel better or have less fatigue. This should be true in the fatigue induced during hypothermia -- the ability to continue work or continue heat production is not furthered by suddenly adding more blood sugar via a candy bar, or even via a sugar injection.

In fact, an article in the April, 1984 edition of *The Physician and Sportsmedicine* reports an experiment which demonstrates that a before activity sugar snack actually DECREASED the ability to perform exercise in their test group. Their group was performing an intermittent high intensity exercise for 2 minutes, followed by a 1 minute rest. This was continued until the subject could no longer perform at approximately 85% of their maximal exercise level. Some subjects were given a 100 gram (3.5 ounce) sugar solution 1 hour prior to exercise, others were given a placebo. Those without the sugar were able to continue 25% longer than those with the sugar.

The spring 1979 edition of *Medical Science and Sports* reported a similar experiment in which 75 grams (2.6 ounces) of sugar was fed to athletes 45 minutes before heavy continuous exercise was performed. Under these conditions, those with the sugar had a 19% decrease in exercise ability.

In a review of the literature which they cite in their *Physician and Sportsmedicine* article, Keller and Schwarzkopf exclaim:

"There is no evidence to demonstrate that a sugar snack taken approximately one hour before exercise is beneficial for subsequent performance. Instead, an increasing body of evidence demonstrates possible harm. Athletes may be well advised to abstain from sugar snacks before exercise."

Why do we frequently feel so much better after having a candy bar when on the trail? I have personally felt this effect many times. Frankly, I believe an equal effect comes from drinking plain water or simply taking a brief rest. The psychological aspect of sports endurance is a tremendous factor in the feeling of fatigue. The individual's attitude has a major impact in how cold they are when it is cold outside also. But attitude alone, no matter how enthused, cannot replace energy substrate required at the muscle cell level. It is in this area that available substrate will make or break the ability of the tissue, and thus the whole person, to perform.

It is becoming apparent that having a high energy carbohydrate snack does not provide energy substrate that will aid increasing exercise tolerance. There is a method of increasing this tolerance, and that is pretrip exercise or training. Training causes an increase in the ability of the cells' enzyme systems to process glucose into muscle glycogen and to utilize this glycogen in producing work or heat energy. There is no easy way around training one's body for work -- and this includes cold stress. Eating a candy bar hoping for some free and easy burst of energy will not provide additional ability to do work or produce heat. In fact, as indicated above, it may actually cause a decrease in the ability to perform sustained maximal work output. I personally do not feel that we need be fearful of a decreased ability to withstand cold from carbohydrate intake. But we should recognize the fact that it will not provide an instant energy substrate that will actually aid in immediately combating heat loss.

It is necessary to consume food substrates to replace the energy which we have consumed through exercise and heat production. While carbohydrate has gotten much of the publicity and study since glucose (a carbohydrate) is an immediate precursor of the high energy substrates, fat and protein are also essential in this process and must be consumed in adequate quantity.

PROTEIN

Shortly after the Persian Wars, an athlete and trainer, Dromeus of Stymphalus -- winner of the long race at Olympia in 456 and 460 BC -- introduced the high protein meat diet. It was erroneously felt that during heavy exercise large losses of protein would be encountered.

This attitude about the necessity of a high protein diet has persisted amongst many athletes, but the following should be noted: (1) Protein is not an efficient energy fuel; (2) The body does not store protein in the sense that it stores fat; (3) Excess protein does not increase strength; and (4) It often takes greater energy to metabolize and digest protein.

The protein intake requirements differ by age, size and sex as indicated in Figure 9. The quantities of protein indicated in this table will be adequate as long as the total calorie requirements are met with adequate amounts of carbohydrate and fat.

However, with regard to protein we are interested in QUALITY as well as QUANTITY. Our muscle structure is composed of protein. Protein, during starvation periods, can also be converted energy. Obviously this is to be avoided as it leads to decrease in strength. It actually provides an inferior source of energy as it provides only 4 kcal of energy per gram, with considerable wastage during its processing (see Specific Dynamic Action of Food).

Proteins consist of building blocks called amino acids. Approximately 20 different amino acids comprise the proteins in our bodies. These amino acids are inter-changeable -- all that is except for eight amino acids that cannot be synthesized by humans. It is important that these 8 amino acids be included in our diet, as it will be the only way we have of acquiring them for incorporation. Protein foods of animal origin contain these essential 8 amino acids in nearly optimal amounts and are thus said to be "high quality proteins."

RECOMMENDED DAILY PROTEIN
REQUIREMENTS BY AGE, SEX, WEIGHT

	Age (years)	Weight (kg) (lbs)		Height (cm) (in)		Energy (kcal)	Protein (g)
Infants	0.0-0.5	6	14	60	24	kg x 117	kg x 2.2
	0.5 - 1.0	9	20	71	28	kg x 108	kg x 2.0
Children	1-3	13	28	86	34	1300	23
	4-6	20	44	110	44	1800	30
	7-10	30	66	135	54	2400	36
Males	11-14	44	97	158	63	2800	44
	15-18	61	134	172	69	3000	54
	19-22	67	147	172	69	3000	54
	23-50	70	154	172	69	2700	56
	51 +	70	154	172	69	2400	56
Females	11-14	44	97	155	62	2400	44
	15-18	54	119	162	65	2100	48
	19-22	58	128	162	65	2100	46
	23-50	58	128	162	65	2000	46
	51 +	58	128	162	65	1800	46
Pregnant						+ 300	+ 30
Lactating						+ 500	+ 20

Reference: *Recommended Dietary Allowances*, 8th rev ed. Food and Nutrition Board, National Research Council - National Academy of Sciences.

FIGURE 9
"RECOMMENDED DAILY PROTEIN REQUIREMENTS BY AGE, SEX, WEIGHT"

FAT

How about a nice slice of blubber? Sounds rather repulsive to our civilized ears, doesn't it? And too bad since fats have a very high food value -- more than twice the food value per weight of carbohydrate or protein. A recent booklet on winter hiking and camping states that it is not essential to include "large amounts" of butter and other fat items in cold weather diets. It states that studies made show there was no indication of fat hunger due to cold. This is, however, contrary to the very point made by the great Arctic explorer, Vilhjalmur Stefansson. A high fat diet was the basis of survival of the Inuit (eskimo). Due to the inadequate intake of fat, Western expedition after expedition died of exposure in the very area that was tolerated by entire families of Inuit. The turning point of High Arctic exploration was made by those explorers who emulated the Inuit diet. But in the modern literature this point is being lost. It was an expensive lesson in the past. In studying the journals of many of these disasters, the turning point seems to occur after the first debilitating year in the field. I have noted on my own trips lasting longer than one month, a considerable desire to increase the fat portion of the diet.

Fats have a calculated food value of 9.45 kcal per gram. For rough calculations, the value 9 kcal per gram is used, thus including a realistic 5% loss in the efficiency of digestion and absorption from the intestines.

SPECIFIC DYNAMIC ACTION OF FOOD

These nutrients not only allow the formation of heat through the work the muscle can perform consuming muscle glycogen, but their very assimilation by the body produces heat. This amounts to a processing energy cost, called "the specific dynamic action of food" (SDA). In other words, the body must expend energy to metabolize these nutrients. And this energy results in heat.

The SDA of food is expressed in the number of kcal required to metabolize that particular nutrient or amount of food. Pure carbohydrates consume 5% of their value during their assimilation. Fats consume 13% and protein 30% of their caloric value to be processed. Most of this energy is released as heat during the two hours after ingestion.

Energy can be spared, and fewer calories eaten, if the basic nutrients are eaten in the proper proportions. That is to say, the specific dynamic action of food is reduced (i.e., the amount of energy wasted to process the food just ingested is reduced) when proper ratios of fat, carbohydrate, and protein are consumed. For example, a mixed diet of protein and carbohydrate consumes 12.5% less calories to process than predicted. A mixed diet of protein and fat consumes 54% less than predicted!

The percentage of fat in the diet, therefore, plays an important role in obtaining more efficiency from the weight of the food consumed. At amounts up to 3,000 kcal, 20 to 25% of the total intake should be fat (66 to 83 grams of fat -- about 3 ounces). At higher caloric values, 30 to 35% should probably come from fat. Of the total grams of fat in the diet, 1% should consist of polyunsaturated oil in order to include the essential fatty acids linoleic and arachidonic acid which aid in proper fat metabolism.

The higher caloric requirements of winter camping can be easily met by increasing fat content of meals by adding cooking oil. This may be added to pancake batter and stews without being noticeable, even by those who do not like fats. The use of butter also makes a palatable addition to the diet.

WINTER ENERGY REQUIREMENTS

In exposure to cold temperatures energy loss is controlled by wearing insulation (clothing), but an increase in total kcal requirement is expected from the type of activity -- many winter projects are physically difficult -- and due to carrying the extra weight of winter clothing. In calculating nutritional requirements for winter camping I have felt that our daily consumption was never over 4,200 kcal. Frequently it was around 3,700 kcal. I have developed these figures both by noting what was consumed during many winter trips into northern Canada and by calculating theoretical energy requirements for work and basal metabolism.

One frequently reads that a winter camping diet will require 6,000 kcal. Very few people are physically conditioned to consume and utilize such an enormous load of food. From personal experience I have never seen a requirement that high. It is possible that conditioned lumberjacks or world class athletes might require such massive calorie amounts, but generally in planning your winter trip, even to the arctic, do not over load your budget or back with unnecessary calories.

Jack Drury, Director of the Wilderness Recreation Leadership program at North Country Community College in Saranac Lake, New York, similarly calculates a maximal requirement of 4,200 kcal for winter camping. He has developed a unique computer program using a VisiCalc spread sheet to assist in generating the itemized food list for both his groups' winter and summer activities. Jack has had many years of experience in the field, both in the west as well as Eastern U.S. to fine tune his nutritional requirement calculations. While this program is still in the developmental phase, he indicates that he is willing to work with others in refining this model and would be interested in corresponding via his office at the college (the Zip Code for Saranac Lake is 12983).

While the higher calorie requirement of winter activity generally means that a larger percentage of fat should be included, there are certain exceptions. At high altitudes, particularly above 16,000 feet (4877 meters), the fat content of the diet should be reduced due to a profound dislike for fats which develops at these elevations. Some persons are affected as low as 15,000 feet (4572 meters). Conversely, sugar is well tolerated at high altitude with two to three times the normal amount being readily consumed in drinks. There is a craving for fresh meat, or highly spiced meat, rather than tinned or freeze-dried foods. But at high altitude it appears that carbohydrates win the taste test over both protein and fat.

WATER

Hydration, or adequate water intake, is extremely important. Natick Army Laboratories have found that a 10% dehydration will cause a 30 to 40% decrease in thermal control. Our water requirements include 800 to 1,000 ml in the urine, 100 ml in stool, and

600 to 1,000 ml as insensible loss through our lungs and skin for a total daily requirement of a minimum of 1,500 ml (1.6 qts.) and up.

A factor predisposing an individual to dehydration is the dry relative humidity under cold weather conditions. All air must be warmed to approximately core temperature and moisture content of this heated air raised to nearly 100% humidity during respiration. If a person is active under these cold, dry conditions, the amount of moisture lost through respiration increases and must be replaced. It is essential to keep up with this loss, with frequent replacement during the day on an hourly basis, if possible.

Thirst lags behind actual water requirements, so water loss must be anticipated and fluid taken before thirst occurs. A useful winter method of ensuring adequate fluid intake is to notice the color of the urine in snow. If it becomes dark and yellow-orange, it is becoming too concentrated and indicates inadequate water intake.

A liter (1.05 quart) heated to 130°F (55°C), about as warm as most people can drink, would provide approximately 18 kcal of heat to a normothermic individual. A liter of water at the freezing point would absorb 37 kcal of energy to heat it to normal core temperature. It is obvious that very warm water cannot replace very many calories, while very cold water can leach a certain number of calories away. There is a thirst quenching aspect of cold water that makes most cold weather travelers crave it. With adequate heat production, the intake of cold water will do no harm. In a hypothermic individual, it would be best to avoid a further calorie drain, but if the choice is between cold water or no water, give the cold water. Water could be warmed by the rescuer with their own body heat to minimize the heat loss, but this heat loss is minimal while the dehydration aspect of this problem is of maximal concern.

We have frequently been warned not to eat snow due to its cooling effect and the harm which it might do us while traveling under cold stress conditions. Popular stories tell us that eating snow is as bad for us as drinking sea water. Snow will leach additional heat from us. The temperature of the snow must be considered, for surface snow will be as cold as the local air temperature, while deeper snow will be as cold as the recent average temperature. If the weather has been -40°F (-40°C), a liter would require 77 kcal of heat to bring it to normal body temperature and an additional 79.7 kcal to melt the ice. This has become a substantial amount of heat loss, in fact 157 kcal. The additional heat consumption to actually melt the ice crystals to liquid water [79.71 kcal per kilogram or liter of water (2.2 pounds or 1.06 quarts)] is called the "latent heat of crystallization" or the "latent heat of fusion."

Snow can be consumed only if there is considerable heat production in a person with good nutrition, who is not fatigued. Snow at a temperature close to the melting point is safer than cold snow with regard to heat loss. Bitter cold snow could do damage by freezing the delicate tissues lining the oral cavity and throat. The old stories are not far from wrong. It is much safer to melt snow prior to consuming it. Adding snow to water already heated will provide more water which, while cooler, will quench the thirst with minimal calorie loss.

You will occasionally read that eating snow will cause dehydration. There is no basis in fact for this statement.

Volitional Exercise

Besides basal metabolic heat generation, the active controlled use of skeletal muscles is a primary method of generating heat. This is the heat produced by hiking, climbing, cutting wood -- in general the purposeful engagement of any outdoor activity. As noted, the basal metabolic rate for the average 155 pound male (70 kg) is approximately 70 kcal per hour. This reflects a basal metabolic rate of 1,700 kcal per day. Skiing x-country uphill at maximal speed on hard snow can generate 18 to 19 kcal/hour (an awesome 1,100 kcal/hour), but this would only be possible for someone who was in world class competition condition, and then for only a limited time.

But even less conditioned individuals can increase their heat production significantly by purposeful exercise. A 180 pound man walking at 2 mph on a hard surface would use 210 kcal/hour, while this work would increase to 828 kcal/hour in soft snow with snow shoes on, if he was able to walk 2.5 mph. Chopping firewood burns 294 kcal/hour during sustained activity. A man in *good physical condition* can sustain a work output up to 630 kcal/hour for long periods of time.

Thus purposeful exercise can not only accomplish an outdoor task, but it provides substantial heat. Figure 10 demonstrates a variety of outdoor tasks and the amount of kcal of heat which these activities generate.

There are limitations to the amount of purposeful exercise that an individual can accomplish. Physical conditioning is the key, as exhaustion -- that is the body's inability to continue muscular activity -- will readily result in hypothermia. The consumption of the energy substrate in the muscle, the muscle glycogen, is the end point of the ability to continue muscular activity. Physical conditioning increases the muscle's ability to replace this essential glycogen store and enhances its ability to utilize it.

This physical conditioning is of utmost importance in preparing for cold stress. There is no easy way around it. A quick trail snack is helpful for morale, but not good enough to provide optimum protection against hypothermia!

The Shivering Response

Another important method of thermogenesis, or heat formation, is shivering. This uncontrolled, rhythmic contraction/relaxation of skeletal muscle is an important emergency measure that the body has to prevent further core heat loss. It is initiated by a cold receptor located in the hypothalamus of the brain, but it works with input from skin sensors, primarily located on the trunk of the body. This remarkable reflex activity causes antagonistic groups of muscle to oscillate at a frequency of 6 to 12 cycles per second.

GROSS ENERGY COSTS FOR DIFFERENT ACTIVITIES OF AVERAGE YOUNG ADULTS

	kcal/min.
Sleep, resting	1.0-1.2
Sitting, at ease, resting	1.5
Sitting, writing, card play	2.1
Standing, at ease	1.7
Dressing, washing	3.0-4.0
Walking, 2 mph, level, hard surface	
100 lb. subject	2.2
140 lb. subject	2.9
160 lb. subject	3.2
180 lb. subject [1]	3.5
Walking 3.5 mph, level, hard surface	
100 lb. subject	3.6
140 lb. subject [2]	4.6
160 lb. subject	5.0
180 lb. subject [3]	5.4
Walking, 4 mph, level, hard surface	
100 lb. subject	4.1
140 lb. subject	5.2
160 lb. subject	5.8
180 lb. subject	6.4
Walking, 4.5 mph, level, hard surface	
155 lb. subject	7.2
Walking, 5 mph, level, hard surface	
155 lb. subject	10.5
Walking, 2 mph, up 15% incline	
155 lb. subject	7.5
Walking, 2 mph, up 25% incline	
155 lb. subject	10.6
Walking, 3 mph, up 5% incline	
155 lb. subject	6.0
Walking, 3 mph, up 10% incline	
155 lb. subject	7.8
Walking, 3 mph, up 15% incline	
155 lb. subject	10.5
Walking, 3.5 mph, up 10% incline	
155 lb. subject	8.9

	kcal/min.
Running, cross country	
140 lb. subject	10.6
Skiing	
level, hard snow, 4 mph	9-10
moderate speed	11-16
uphill, hard snow, max speed	18-19
Climbing, slope 1 in 5.7 grade	
180 lb. subject	
with 11 lb. load	10.7
with 22 lb. load	11.6
with 44 lb. load	12.2
Canoeing	
2.5 mph	3.0
4.0 mph	7.0
Cycling	
5.5 mph	4.5
9.4 mph	7.0
13.1 mph	11.1
Breaking firewood	4.9
Driving a car	2.8
Driving a motorcycle	3.4
Volleyball	3.5
Tennis	7.1
Swimming	
Back stroke	
25 yd./min.	5.0
30 yd./min.	7.0
35 yd./min.	9.0
40 yd./min.	11.0
Breast stroke	
40 yd./min.	10.0
Side stroke	
40 yd./min.	11.0
Climbing, slope 1 in 4.7 grade	
180 lb. subject	
with 11 lb load	12.1
with 22 lb load	12.7
with 44 lb load	13.2

NOTE 1.   At 2.5 mph a 180 lb subject would increase work to 13.8 on soft snow with snow shoes; with 44 lb. load 20.2

NOTE 2.   At 3.5 mph a 140 lb subject would increase work to 5.6 on level grass, 6.2 on stubble field, 7 on ploughed field

NOTE 3.   At 3.5 mph a 180 lb subject would increase work to 11.9 on hard snow

NOTE 4.   When markedly rough, slower speed will compensate for surface difference

NOTE 5.   Walking down a 10% decline at various speeds will result in up to 25% less energy requirement than level surface; very steep decline will increase work above level surface - no figures available

NOTE 6.   Canoe data for moderately skilled subjects, favorable weather, average of 4 trials for this data

NOTE 7.   Wide tires add 1 kcal/min. for all speeds

Adapted from Passmore, R., and Durnin, J. V. G. A.: Human Energy Expenditure. Physiol. Rev., 35:801-840, 1955

FIGURE 10   "GROSS ENERGY COSTS FOR DIFFERENT ACTIVITIES OF AVERAGE YOUNG ADULTS"

In the hierarchy of maintaining body heat, shivering plays both important stop-gap and fine tuning roles. If we have not provided adequate additional heat, if we have not added enough insulation to our clothing, if purposeful muscle activity has not provided adequate additional heat, and if the body's various heat preservation reflexes have not kept the core temperature above 97°F (36°C), shivering will result.

An initial shiver in a warm person may also result from sudden cooling of the skin or inhalation of cold air, thus providing a rapid warming function. This "early shiver response" helps establish other reflex mechanisms to protect the core temperature and does not represent a dropping core temperature.

Shivering can increase heat production by about 4.5 times the resting rate of heat production to 500 kcal per hour. But at a price. It is a highly inefficient method of heat production. While shivering the body is willing to squander remaining energy stores, totally depleting muscle glycogen stores and energy substrates available to it in the desperate attempt to keep core temperature from falling further.

If core temperature remains depressed, shivering will continue -- if the core temperature raises, it will stop. Shivering will also stop if the energy substrate "runs out." At that point a precipitous drop in core temperature will occur. The violent shiver is the body's last serious defense against sliding into potentially lethal deep hypothermia.

In case of rapid heat loss, such as in cold water immersion hypothermia, depression of the core temperature can occur to the point that shivering ceases even though energy substrate is still available. Evidence indicates that this suppression of the shiver reflex probably occurs at 86°F (30°C). It appears that alcohol suppresses the shiver reflex. The fact that these victims have not exhausted energy substrate stores, may affect their ability to survive when they are reheated -- although many other factors are also important when examining the differences between a slow onset or chronic hypothermia and a rapid onset, or acute immersion hypothermia.

Besides being an inefficient use of valuable energy stores, the shiver response causes an increased blood flow to muscles and therefore pulls blood from the body core. This increased circulation causes a loss of insulation and increases heat loss by about 25%.

A few other facts should be mentioned concerning the very valuable shiver response. First, some people do not have a shiver response, and in others the ability to shiver is diminished. And

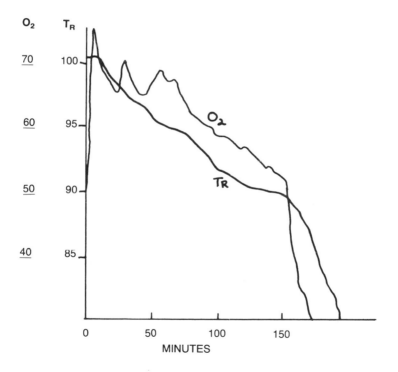

FIGURE 11.   "GRAPH ILLUSTRATING SUDDEN LOSS OF CORE TEMPERATURE
AFTER CONSUMPTION OF ENERGY SUBSTRATE"
The rectal temperature curve (T_r) in this subject makes a sudden downward plunge at about the 90 degree Fahrenheit (32.2°C) point. As an indicator that this is due to the loss of energy substrate, it will be noted that the oxygen consumption (O_2), which indicates the amount of energy substrate being used, and therefore available for use, has dropped simultaneously. In this graph, the oxygen consumption is in units of ml/kg/min. and the temperature curve in Fahrenheit degrees. Source: Marlin Kreider M.D. in *Appalachia*, Dec. 1980.

second, do not be overly afraid of shivering. It is a useful method of fine tuning the body heat production and it does not mean that one is in imminent danger of hypothermia. A greater danger than shivering is the feeling of exhaustion.

While shivering will rapidly lead to exhaustion, it is easy to see that an exhausted person will have a decreased or no ability to shiver. Thus, exhaustion by itself strips away this valuable last-ditch defense mechanism of the body. In order to properly tolerate exposure to hypothermia conditions, we must strive NOT to become exhausted and NOT to have to rely on shivering to maintain our core temperature. We must use whatever intellect we have available to counter further heat loss and otherwise improve our chances of survival at this moment. A further decrease in core temperature will certainly occur when substrates have been exhausted. This core decrease will subsequently depress our mental ability to cope properly with this emergency situation.

We have been warned in the lore of the north not to dare stop and rest lest we fail to awaken and freeze to death. I traveled north with a person once who had just read *CALL OF THE WILD*. It was virtually impossible to get that person to agree to a rest stop due to the fear of freezing to death. But maintaining a reserve of that precious muscle glycogen and minimizing the general level of fatigue are critical factors in assuring our survival in a cold stress situation. All of the factors causing fatigue are not fully understood, but it is without a doubt a warning of imminent exhaustion. This exhaustion must not be allowed to occur, because with it we lose the ability to do work or to shiver -- both of the major body functions which produce heat to prevent hypothermia. Even with adequate insulation, exhaustion may easily allow hypothermia to develop.

In this section I have tackled two popular myths. First, that one should keep going, lest one freeze to death. The other, eat candy for instant energy for continued work and prevention of hypothermia. Scientific evidence demonstrates that both of these techniques are faulty. Rest is important. The cold exposed individual should rest to prevent exhaustion. He should also eat to prevent total loss of energy substrate. But this eating is best done during the rest periods, the energy acquired from it will be slow in coming and will be dependent upon prior physical conditioning as to how fast it will replenish the muscle glycogen stores.

A sensible approach to enjoying a safe prolonged exposure to hypothermic conditions is:

1. Proper pretrip physical conditioning
2. Proper pretrip nutritional status
3. Proper dress
4. Adequate rest during the trip
5. Eating adequately to replenish energy stores while on the trip
6. Adequate hydration while on the trip

4.   HANDLING THE COLD

The Physiological Preservation of Heat

The human response to cold stress takes many forms. Some are an important means of conserving or replacing lost body heat, while other responses are minor. Various other mammals have methods of protection available to them that are either rudimentary or missing in humans. And, there are frequently detrimental side effects from many of the physiological responses that are meant to protect us from a lowering core temperature.

These responses, and their importance to the maintenance of life, can vary with the rapidity of cold stress onset, severity of the environment, physiology of the individual, and are influenced by underlying medical conditions, drug or alcohol intake, age, sex, and degree of physical conditioning.

Our attempts to aid these responses in conserving heat loss, or maximizing their ability to produce heat, is important in developing intelligent field approaches to the prevention or correction of hypothermia.

Vascular Control of Thermoregulation

An interesting aspect of body heat control is that 95% of the heat produced daily by the body must be removed. Yet, under exposure to a cold environment a mechanism must be available to decrease this remarkable heat loss.

For thermoregulation purposes the body may be considered to be constructed in two zones: the inner core and an exterior mantle. Heat is constantly being produced internally by the basal metabolic activity of the organ systems, by the specific dynamic action of food, and by muscular contraction. The first two mentioned are core produced, while muscle activity is the inner mantle region -- the outer mantle consists of the skin and subcutaneous fat layer.

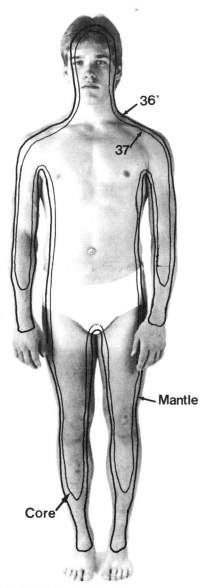

FIGURE 12   "A NORMO-THERMIC INDIVIDUAL"
The above figure has a large, warm core with a thin mantle, thus allowing maximal heat loss to the environment.

Body fluids, fat, and muscle are good thermal insulators and poor conductors. A 1 centimeter (.4 inch) thick piece of perfused muscle is as good an insulator as a 1 centimeter thick piece of cork (conductivity = 18 kcal/hour/°C gradient). A man at rest produces about 72 kcal of heat per hour. The amount of heat conductance from the core to the mantle will equal from 5 to 10 kcal per degree Celsius gradient per hour. With the amount of insulation present in his mantle, only 20 to 40 kcal per hour of heat could be transported to the surface, depending upon the temperature gradient. Internal heat cannot, therefore be readily eliminated by conductance.

The majority of internal heat is eliminated by forced convection in which warm blood from the interior is carried to the cooler surface of the mantle by the circulating blood. The skin has remarkable properties allowing extensive regulation of blood flow, both from local factors and central nervous system control. This blood flow can range from 30 ml/minute (.5% of cardiac output) under cold stress conditions, to 300 ml/minute (5% of cardiac output) under normal temperature conditions, to 3000 ml/minute during times of high heat stress. There are two major components in this change of blood flow that play enormous roles in the rate of heat transfer. One is vasoconstriction, the other vasodilation.

The process of vasodilation can increase blood flow to the outer skin surface, the epidermis, by 100 fold, thus increasing heat loss by as much as 20-fold. Similarly, vasoconstriction can effectively increase the insulating depth of the outer mantle, by decreasing blood flow.

Linkages of outer blood veins, which carry the cooler blood back to the core, and sets of deep veins, are responsible for considerable heat conservation. The deep veins travel in a neurovascular bundle, the importance of which is their close proximity to the artery carrying warmer blood outward to the extremity. Under cold stress there is a shift in venous blood from the outer veins to these inner veins. This allows a conductive heat exchange between the cool blood flowing back and the warm blood flowing outward. This is called the countercurrent heat exchange. Cool venous blood is

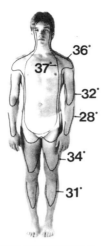

FIGURE 13 "A COLD-STRESSED INDIVIDUAL"

The above figure shows the shrinking zone of core temperature with a larger, cooler mantle formation. This provides a greater insulation layer from cold, yet it means a decreased total heat store.

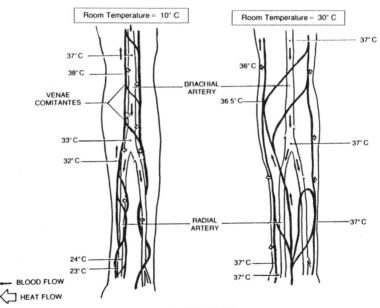

FIGURE 14 "COUNTER-CURRENT HEAT EXCHANGE"

During heat stress and under most normal temperature conditions, the surface veins return most of the blood from the extremities, as illustrated in the arm on the left, above. During cold stress, the blood is returned to the core along veins that lie deep, next to the major arteries. This decreases cooling on the return, and allows an exchange of heat between the artery and vein which is described in the text.

warmed as it returns to the core and arterial blood is cooled as it travels away from the core. Blood circulation to the extremities continues, while heat loss is minimized, since heat is not carried away by this flow. In times of heat stress, the returning venous blood is carried primarily by the surface veins and away from the warm arterial heat source, thus preventing the returning cooler blood from being heated by the hot arterial blood.

These vasoconstrictor and blood flow shifts are so effective that upon exposure to cold, a rise of the core temperature of .9°F (.5°C) occurs. This decrease in circulation effectively increases the mantle depth and decreases the core size, thus providing a greater depth of insulation to the core. This will result in a lower skin temperature and the loss of some heat stores during the initial cold response.

It is easy to glide over a statement such as "loss of some heat stores" without realizing its significance. This means that the total amount of heat in the body will be allowed to decrease as the mass of tissue in the smaller core attempts to remain warm and the mantle becomes larger and is allowed to become cooler. The body gives up trying to heat its entire mass and by simply maintaining the smaller interior core near normal temperature, the total amount of heat in the body (which can be computed by multiplying mass times temperature) has decreased. This fact is particularly important in rescue work, when we need to consider the total amount of heat required to rewarm a victim, or in considering the amount of heat which a rescuer may be able to provide with his own body.

Other Physiologic Responses to Cold Stress

Pilo-erection is a major response in birds and some mammals to cold stress. In man, no matter how hairy, this results only in "goose bumps" with no significant increase in insulation.

In the human male a cremasteric reflex causes the scrotum to shrink, pulling the testes close to the pelvis. While insignificant as a heat loss prevention technique, it is important in protecting the testes from deleterious cold. The male scrotum is a heat exchange mechanism, designed to keep the testes at a temperature lower than the core. This is essential, not only for the proper production of sperm, but also it is known that an increase incidence of testicular tumors can occur if the testes are retained within the abdominal cavity, probably due to the higher temperature in that area.

In sudden exposure to cold water in immersion or acute hypothermia, a gasp reflex can occur. This seems to be related to spasm of the diaphragm and can result in a sudden sucking in of air which could result in drowning. The gasp reflex is not an isolated spasm, but a series of contractures which make breathing difficult until these spasms are relaxed by both mental and physiological control. These spasms generally cease after a 10 to 15 minute immersion time.

A reflex which has received considerable reporting in the press is the "mammalian diving reflex." This can occur in youngsters, and is probably most active up to at least the age of 2 or 3. It amounts to a sudden reflex slowing of breathing, heart rate, and a rapid cooling of body temperature together with a loss of consciousness. The most important aspect of this reflex is that blood and oxygen is selectively shunted from the lungs and heart to the brain. This small but vital oxygen rich blood flow protects this organ until the body cools sufficiently to lower the metabolism and oxygen requirements. It is possible for an acute cold water immersion victim to be rescued after 30 minutes of submersion and have no brain damage after resuscitation. This reflex is a rare exception rather than the rule, but the fact that it exists points out how important it is to make every attempt at resuscitation in a "cold victim" even after prolonged submersion. In fact there is a dictum that "NO HYPOTHERMIA VICTIM IS TO BE CONSIDERED DEAD, UNLESS THEY ARE WARM AND DEAD." The importance of applying this to the near drowning victim is to recognize the possibility that hypothermia may have protected such a victim from brain damage, even though they have been submerged longer than 10 minutes.

Immersion in water colder than 68°F (20°C) can result in hypothermia. The mammalian diving reflex, however, seems limited to acute submersion in very cold water, and is found almost exclusively in children under 5 years of age. Cold water submersion, particularly in youngsters, can result in such rapid cooling of the body, that resuscitation is possible even without the mammalian diving reflex. Several studies seemed to indicate, however, that the lower the child's temperature upon admission to the emergency room, the poorer the chance of recovery without brain damage. This was probably due to the fact that a very low body temperature generally meant longer submersion times. (See section on Submersion Hypothermia, page 76.)

As the core temperature decreases, certain physiological changes are simultaneously occurring. As mentioned, one is the literal formation of a larger, cooler mantle and a shrinking core. Blood circulation to this exterior mantle has been decreased and shunted to the core. This results in a fluid overload which must be corrected. The kidney response is to dump some of this fluid, a process called "cold diuresis."

Various components of the blood such as the blood sugar, electrolytes (sodium, potassium, and chloride particularly), metabolic by-products from the fatigue of exercise or shivering, and the blood cells themselves are affected by this concentrating of the blood volume in the shrinking core and by the further cooling of this core.

The degree of each of these changes cannot be predicted by the temperature of the victim, by the rapidity of onset of hypothermia, or by any other parameter. This uncertainty of the metabolic status makes the medical management of hypothermia an individualized problem and a cookbook approach to the proper emergency room treatment cannot be blindly followed.

But, we can take advantage of several aspects of the individual's change in response to this cold stress in our approach to the hypothermic victim in the field.

One of the major consequences of hypothermia is the decrease in the basal metabolic rate. At 82.4°F (28°C) it falls to 50% of its normal level. This results in a lower requirement for oxygen by the body's cells and, in fact, a decreased requirement for energy substrates such as muscle glycogen, glucose, and fatty acids, with less production of waste products.

Under the conditions of severe hypothermia the oxygen will not break its binding to hemoglobin as well and therefore will not be as readily available for use by the body cells. The blood is thicker and will not flow as easily. The heart beats slower. Fortunately the decreased requirement for oxygen protects the cells from death by anoxia or lack of oxygen.

Similarly other body functions are slowed to the point of protection. Dr. William Mills, Anchorage, Alaska, has called this protection while in a hypothermic state being in a "metabolic icebox." Once rewarming is started, the protection of the suspended animation of the "metabolic icebox" is lost. The dehydration, changes in acid-base balance of the blood, imbalances of sugar, potassium and other electrolytes, blood clotting mechanism, oxygenation of tissues and removal of waste products -- all become unstable. If the rewarming occurs rapidly, the values necessary for safe recovery change rapidly and must be corrected just as fast as they occur. It is the loss of metabolic control during the rewarming process which causes death in the rescued victim.

Physiological Contributions to Heat Loss

In addition to the physical laws which govern heat exchange there are certain physiological actions which contribute directly to heat loss.

RESPIRATION HEAT LOSS

Maintenance of life requires respiration primarily for oxygen exchange. Activity of any kind increases the rate or depth of respiration. Cold air must be warmed and humidity increased by the upper airways of the nose, the nasal and oral pharynx, to 100% humidity and virtually core temperature to prevent drying and cold vasospasm of bronchial and lung tissue.

HEAT LOSS DURING RESPIRATION

Air Temperature	Convective Heat Loss For Average Man kcal/hour	
68°F (20°C)	5.8	
32°F (0°C)	12.5	Add 24.3 kcal/hour
-4°F (-20°C)	19.3	Evaporative heat loss
-40°F (-40°C)	26.	

Convective heat loss from warming air varies directly with the outside air temperature. The evaporative heat loss of respiration is a steady loss of 24.3 kcal/hour, which is independent of temperature and which must be added to the above figures.

FIGURE 15   "HEAT LOSS DURING RESPIRATION"

The evaporative heat loss from providing humidity to expired air, varies with the relative humidity of the outside air and the rate of respiration. Assuming a respiratory rate of 1.4 kg of air per hour, at temperatures below freezing the rather dry relative humidity remains constant for this calculation and would result in a fairly steady heat loss of 24.3 kcal/hour. This amount of energy loss should be added to the above table to determine the total heat loss due to respiration.

This air has been heated and humidity increased at a cost and when expelled it represents a source of lost body heat. This mechanism is so important in some mammals that it represents their primary method of cooling the body during heat stress -- for example, the panting dog.

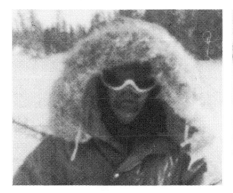

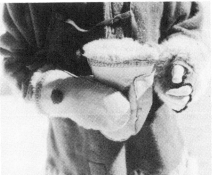

FIGURE 16A "FUR HOOD - SNORKEL FOR WINTER WEAR"
The fur trimmed hood acts as a snorkel to allow re-breathing warmed and humidified air during cold weather exposure. Photo by the author in Northern Manitoba.

FIGURE 16B "FUR TRIMMED PARKA SLEEVE AND MITTEN PLUG TECHNIQUE"
The above photo shows a fur trimmed sleeve and a mitten with an interior trim of fur, used to make a draft-free plug without the use of constricting elastic or draw strings. The photo, taken by the author, shows the great wilderness author Calvin Rutstrum demonstrating his method in 1977.

BELLOWS EFFECT

Movement of an individual will increase convection loss. But movement also produces the "bellows effect." This phenomenon is familiar to all winter campers. The slightest movement in a sleeping bag briefly blows hot air out and sucks cold air in. This movement also allows heat loss from parkas. To compensate for this, manufacturers tend to place elastic wrist cuffs in garments. In cold weather camping any restriction of peripheral blood flow increases the chance of frost bite. To avoid this problem the Inuit (eskimo) placed a fur rim around the edge of parka sleeves and also attached a fur inner cuff to the heavy mittens (see Figure 16B). They could thus place their hands easily into mittens, which were attached from a cord that hung out their sleeves, the fur plugging any air movement with no restriction of blood flow.

The parka bellows effect around the neck is generally decreased in bulky garments due to their tight fit on the upper torso and at the shoulders.

A fur trimmed hood on a parka can form a breathing tunnel, or snorkel, for cold weather use that will reduce the bellows effect, prevent much direct wind conduction loss, decrease respiration heat losses, and block radiation loss from the head. Any parka designed for serious winter use must have a generous hood, preferably with a frost resistant trim.

If a major blood vessel were to come close to the skin, it would be in danger of allowing unnecessary heat loss during bitter cold conditions. The Inuit apparently knew of the importance of the femoral artery which travels from deep in the abdomen to relatively near the surface of the front aspect of the leg beneath the inguinal ligaments (see Figure 17). It is for this reason that they developed the short outer pants which provide additional thermal protection to this vital artery. These pants could easily be removed, since they were worn over their trousers and were large enough to easily slip over foot wear.

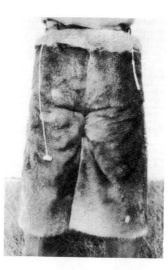

FIGURE 17   "INUIT SHORT
OUTER PANTS"
These outer pants made of caribou (shown
here) or seal skin were used by the Inuit
(eskimo) to provide additional thermal protection to the femoral arteries and groin during extreme cold stress.

URINARY HEAT LOSS

Urinating seems an awful waste of body heat, but a quick calculation demonstrates that this loss is not significant. The average urinary output per day is approximately 1500 ml (1.6 quarts). It takes 55½ kcal to heat that quantity of water from freezing to body core temperature. Water drunk warmer would cause less of a heat loss, but the unusual aspect of cold weather travel is the tremendous desire for a very cold drink of water. Due to this rather low energy requirement, drinking cold water is not a harmful technique for winter travel in the healthy individual. See a full discussion of this subject on page 29.

SHIVER HEAT LOSS

As mentioned elsewhere, shivering is a primary method of increasing heat production in the body. However, this activity causes increased blood flow to muscle mass, vasodilation, and an increase in potential bellows effect. Shivering results in a 25% increase in body heat loss. As shivering can increase heat production between 200 to 700%, it is still a valuable heat generating technique. But minimizing potential losses during the shivering process can make it more valuable.

COLD INDUCED VASODILATION HEAT LOSS

A method of preventing frostbite is a periodic expansion (vasodilation) of the arteries. This carries the fancy term "cold induced vasodilation," but is frequently called the "hunting response." At a tissue temperature of 59°F (15°C) vasoconstriction will be maximal. If the tissue cools further to 50°F (10°C), intermittent periods of vasodilation occur to apparently provide some protection to tissues from frostbite. This however does allow a heat loss. The body has sacrificed a portion of the heat preservation aspect of vasoconstriction to preserve the life of the tissues involved. Periodic vasodilation is an insignificant source of heat loss.

Most physiological responses of the body are to preserve or generate heat, not to allow loss. The physiological losses mentioned here are basically a trade off. The increased heat loss caused by shivering is far outweighed by the amount of heat generated; the loss of heat from countercurrent heat exchange is important to the preservation of warmer returning blood to the core; periodic vasodilation to prevent frostbite causes a very small calorie loss compared to the enormous contribution of vasoconstriction to heat preservation.

5. TREATMENT OF HYPOTHERMIA
Field Diagnosis of Hypothermia

In 1866 Sir Clifford Allbutt refined Galileo's invention, the thermometer, for clinical use. The commonly available clinical thermometer used today has a temperature range of 96°F (35.5°C) to 106°F (41.1°C). Hypothermia is generally defined as a core temperature below 95°F (35°C). The routinely used clinical thermometer is wholly inadequate to evaluate a hypothermic state. As will be noted shortly victims with a core temperature below 90°F (32.2°C) must be treated quite differently in the hospital than those with temperatures above this point. There are specific thermometers made for low temperature readings. While several of these are on the market, a very low reading thermometer is available from Indiana Camp Supply.

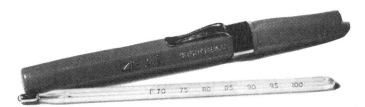

FIGURE 18 "HYPOTHERMIA THERMOMETER"
Most clinical thermometers will not read below 94°F (34.4°C). The above imported thermometer reads as low as 70°F (21.1°C). Available from Indiana Camp Supply, Box 344F, Pittsboro, IN 46167, (Phone 317/892-3310).

The hypothermia, or low reading thermometer, must be used rectally to provide a valid result. This obviously is impractical under most field situations. One must generally rely on symptoms to make the diagnosis, but these symptoms have proven consistently unreliable (see Figure 1, page 4). The urgency in being able to recognize this condition stems not only from the necessity of treating it, but also involves a recognition of the loss of mental ability that is part of the hypothermic syndrome. Hypothermia will not occur unless an unexpected event has taken place. The party is in trouble, perhaps not severely so, but never-the-less in trouble. Accurate assessments of the situation and plans of action must be made and continuously updated.

What if the leader or key persons in the party become hypothermic? A major aspect of the illness, hypothermia, is the loss of mental reasoning. This can be insidious. Both the leaders and their companions may scarcely be aware of their diminishing senses. Whenever a group is in trouble strong leadership is essential. One does not want to advocate any method whereby the fabric of leadership may be constantly challenged, particularly during times of extreme stress and danger. Those are the very times when leadership should remain inviolate and generally unchallenged.

The method of challenge I would advocate is the old "walking the straight line" technique. This is a test for cerebellar ataxia and it is a fairly reliable indication of a decrease in cerebellar, and thus general brain function. While ataxia is a motor coordination skill, it indicates that the brain has become hypothermic to the point that its logical and memory functions are also probably impaired. In this test, upon challenge from one's peers or in response to self testing, simply attempt to walk straddling a straight line for a distance of 10 yards (9 meters). If this proves difficult or impossible, then the party must make immediate provisions to allow the least affected member to assume leadership (providing they would otherwise be capable) to immediately extract the group from the continued effects of the inclement weather.

Many people who succumb to hypothermia are solitary travelers, but many are not. Early in my career of leading groups into the bush I thought ill of the group leader -- or the members of a group -- who would allow a solitary member to die of hypothermia. I felt it should be all or none; that it was incredible to imagine allowing a trip partner to freeze to death without somehow redistributing clothing, huddling in bags together, doing whatever was necessary to keep all members of the party alive.

I now realize that this concept was idealistic, but not realistic. There are many reasons why a single member of a party might die while others live. The physical conditioning of the individual is preeminent in predicting survival under cold stress, as are mental attitude, equipment, concurrent illness, nutritional status, extent of exertion, level of fatigue, and degree of exposure differences various party members might experience on a particular trip.

It is not an uncommon event to hear of an entire group experiencing signs or symptoms of hypothermia -- after all, their degree of exposure has been similar and may be beyond what they anticipated with their clothing. But because of these differences in individual well being, it would be rather unusual for an entire group (not including immersion accidents) to suddenly experience hypothermia. Generally a luckless member of the group will become the early warning system for his companions. Techniques of spotting group hypothermia danger should generally monitor each member, but particular attention should be paid to the most fatigued, least conditioned, or most poorly equipped individual. Changes in personality are possible clues of fatigue and forewarner of hypothermia development.

There have been reports in newspapers of entire groups becoming hypothermic, virtually at once. Naturally, groups exposed to sudden changes in weather conditions could result in mass hypothermia casualties. However, one must also consider the phenomenon of group hysteria when dealing with multiple cases from a group where members succumbed virtually simultaneously. When confronted with such mass casualties, it is mandatory to take temperatures with an adequate low reading thermometer to rule out hypothermia rather than relying upon symptoms.

REPLACING LOST HEAT
The Caloric Deficit and Its Replacement

Severely hypothermic individuals have depleted their caloric reserve, depressing their core temperature below 90°F (32°C), and have a caloric debt of about 500 kcal. It takes about 60 kcal to rewarm the patient one degree Fahrenheit.

HEAT REPLACEMENT BY FLUIDS

A liter (1.05 quart) of intravenous solution which has been heated to 110°F (43.3°C), which is about as warm as it can be given, would contribute 17 kcal.

The chronic hypothermia victim IS in a dehydrated state. In fact a deficit of 5.5 liters (5.8 quarts) exists, pulled mostly from the interstitial tissue, some from cell fluids, and the rest from the vascular system. The resuscitation of these individuals will require replacing this fluid, but the control of electrolytes, blood sugar, and acid-base balance will limit the rate of the I.V. therapy. If the entire 5.5 liters of warmed fluid were infused, it would replace only a little over 90 kcal to a person who requires 500 kcal to be brought back to normal core temperature. The use of heated I.V. fluids in the wilderness situation is, of course, impractical.

If the victim is conscious, warm fluids may be given by mouth. But as can be guessed from the above, the amount of heat actually provided to the victim is very small. If the core temperature is 90°F (32°C), a quart of fluid heated to 140°F (65°C) will provide only 30 kcal of heat to a person who is depleted by 500 kcal. And the amount of heated fluid that the victim will be able to intake is obviously limited.

When hot fluids are given by mouth, it is possible for a pharyngeal reflex to occur which initiates vasodilation, thus increasing the blood flow to the skin and the extremities. This in turn could cause a core cooling that may surpass the meager amount of heat provided by the oral intake. The hypothermic victim must be provided adequate insulation so that a vasodilation will not expose this warmed surface blood to low ambient temperature and cause further blood cooling. A core cooling may result from this shunting of blood regardless. There is some concern about a possible irritability of the heart, also caused by the pharyngeal reflex, with the possible initiation of a ventricular fibrillation of the heart. Probably, in the conscious victim, protected from further heat loss, the above detrimental problems are minimal. The gradual addition of heat from warm fluids will be a welcome psychological boost to the victim, even if the physiological benefit is minimal.

A method of providing large volumes of heated fluid, readily available in most emergency rooms, is the technique of peritoneal dialysis. Using sterile technique, special catheters are inserted into the abdominal cavity, taking care not to penetrate the intestines or other vital organs. With this method a liter of fluid is flushed through the abdominal cavity with a starting temperature of 110.3°F (43.5°C). Since the abdominal organs receive 25% of the cardiac output under resting condition, bathing them in warm fluid provides adequate contact with the core circulation. At a flow rate of 5 liters per hour, the patient will obtain 85 kcal/hour. Tight medical control of the content and temperature of these solutions and of the patient must be maintained during this procedure. The benefits of the technique, besides availability in most emergency rooms, is that it provides heat without fluid overload. It also is a useful technique to remove many drugs that urban hypothermic victims have been taking, which is frequently a cause for their spending the night outside and becoming hypothermic in the first place.

HEAT REPLACEMENT BY INHALED AIR

The use of heated, humidified oxygen has been advocated to assist in the rewarming process. Heated, humidified oxygen can be tolerated as warm as 116°F (47°C), but it is generally administered at about 104°F (40°C). The amount of heat which this technique can replace is rather small. It is directly related to the rate and volume of breathing. At a total volume of 3 liters/minute the patient will gain 9.4 kcal/hour, while at 10 liters/minute the heat gain will be 23.7 kcal/hour. The normal tidal volume, or amount of air that is breathed in and out, approaches the 10 liter/minute figure. Respirations will be decreased in a hypothermic individual to the point that a normal tidal volume will not be reached.

To increase the amount of heat provided by heated, humidified oxygen, the patient can be intubated -- that is a tube placed into the trachea or windpipe, and the breathing rate and depth controlled by a respirator. Achieving maximum settings with this equipment would generally allow an inspired air temperature of 113°F (45°C) with a total tidal volume of 20 liters/minute. If the patient had a core temperature of 82.4°F (28°C), there could be a calculated heat gain of 46 kcal/hour. If this were the only source of additional heat for the victim, even at this maximal rate this technique would allow a temperature increase of less than 1°F (.5°C) per hour.

While the technology to produce heated air with light weight equipment in the field is possible, as noted above the actual heat gain by the victim, even with intubation, is minimal. The most important aspect of providing heated air in any setting is that at least a further heat loss via respiration is NOT occurring. Buddy breathing has been mentioned in the literature as possibly of some benefit. This amounts to a variation of respiratory resuscitation. Rather than breathing for the victim, the rescuer simply breaths along with the victim using standard mouth-to-mouth positioning. This is not practical during most rescue situations, and as noted above, the heat gain is minimal. An easier approach in the field is simply to avoid further heat loss by having the victim rebreathe his own air through a wool scarf, etc. If the victim is placed with a rescuer in a sleeping bag positioning both of the heads beneath the bag outlet salvages the respiratory heat and provides a souce of heated, humidified air.

HEAT REPLACEMENT BY RADIATION

Radiant heat is a source of heat which we often utilize, frequently without realizing it. Heat from the infrared spectrum of sun light provides a direct source of warmth. Since it is highly reflective, snow, water, and sand increase this radiant heat source considerably. On even cold days, particularly in areas sheltered from wind currents, the warmth of the sun can be a pleasant sensation.

The use of a reflecting fire, a standard technique in the old woodcraft days, was worth the effort of construction due to the amount of heat reflected forward from the fire providing warmth for the fireside observer as well as the cook pot or spit (Figure 19).

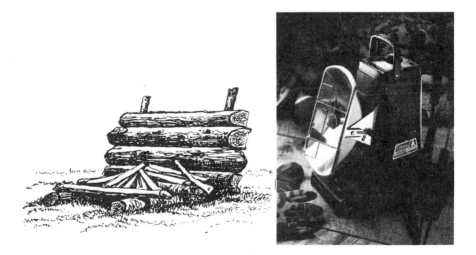

FIGURE 19   "THE REFLECTING FIRE"
The traditional method of building a wood reflecting fire, this technique provides a substantial increase in the amount of heat directed forward.

FIGURE 20   "THE RADIANT HEATER"
A modern version of a portable radiant heating technique is the radiant heater.

Producing a hollow in the snow to protect from wind, and aid in reflection of heat from the sun or external fire source; the use of metallized plastic sheeting for heat gathering (as opposed to its general use as a wrap to aid in radiant heat loss -- see page 102); the use of infrared heat sources (Figure 20 a Coleman type radiant heater); and the use of radiant energy from heated stones and stoves, are all methods of adding heat via radiant energy. The use of radiant heat can be helpful in select circumstances when treating hypothermia, but it should never be used for thawing frostbite victims. It must be cautiously used whenever the skin is numb from cold, for radiation heat from close sources can easily result in burns.

HEAT REPLACEMENT BY CONDUCTION

Conductive heat sources must be carefully utilized or burns may result. Placing a warm rock against the victim is a conductive heat transfer, while placing it near him would be a safer, yet less intense, radiant heat transfer. Conduction can cause burns, particularly when the victim is unconscious or his skin is numb. Conduction of heat through cloth, such as huddled, clothed rescuers or wrapped warm objects, is safer yet a less intense heat source.

The immersion of the victim in warm water is an example of a profound method of initiating rapid heat transfer. Indeed, this is the method of choice, when available, for the acute hypothermic victim. It may be safely used for the chronic hypothermia patient only if the rescuers are capable of maintaining tight metabolic control as the rapid increase in body temperature will result in major alterations of blood flow, glucose, electrolyte, and other metabolic patterns.[1]

This means that for chronic hypothermia it is a potentially dangerous method and should be avoided in the wilderness setting. The amount of heat, and the speed by which it may be transferred

[1]The blood levels for these items must be determined and adjusted every 15 minutes if hot water immersion is to be ''safely'' used.

with this technique, is remarkable. There is probably no faster method other than the sophisticated cardio-pulmonary bypass machine used in the operating room. It can be as tricky and as dangerous to use.

HEAT REPLACEMENT BY CONVECTION

Warm air currents provide heat via convection. Generally, the use of warm air currents to replace heat is not a practical technique for rescue work. It supposes that air can be heated and forced past the victim. If the victim is damp, this method will result in an evaporative heat loss so every precaution should be made to dry the subject thoroughly. If the air is warm enough, the consumption of energy to allow the evaporation of water from damp clothing will come from the hot air and not from the victim's diminished heat stores. Because of this, with an adequate amount of warm air it is safe to dry and warm the victim simultaneously. Care must be taken not to cause burns in vulnerable, numb skin using convection reheating techniques.

Field Management of Chronic Hypothermia

MANAGEMENT OF IMPENDING MILD HYPOTHERMIA
When active, ventilate excess heat

It is perfectly proper, in fact necessary, to ventilate excess heat to the environment. If your activity level is high enough to produce sweating, it must be avoided by allowing cold air contact with the under layers of your winter outfit, or even with your skin. Opening parkas, removing mittens, taking one's hat off -- whatever is necessary to prevent overheating.

When tired, preserve heat

When one feels exhaustion developing, or otherwise knows that their physical limitations are being reached, it will be necessary to slow down the rate of energy loss. You will have to do less work, which means less heat will be produced. At this point it will be necessary to avoid as much heat loss to the environment as possible.

Keep clothing dry

Every effort should be made to have dry clothing on. Jackets should be closed, hats and mittens donned, and hoods raised if they are available. If a member of the party is reaching exhaustion, they should be provided the clothing to prevent heat loss. If jackets are not adequate to prevent cold penetration (which means a heat loss is occurring), shelter from wind must be sought.

Replace wet clothing

Wet clothing must be replaced. Regardless of fabric, wet clothing will not insulate as well as dry. Using the new synthetics will minimize heat loss if the garment is wet, but they will not prevent loss of heat from the latent heat of vaporization. Remember, it will take 245 kcal of heat to evaporate 1 pound (.45 kilograms) of water. As wet clothing can be carrying several pounds of water, the importance of preventing further heat loss due to evaporation is apparent.

Cover, insulate wet clothing

If the wet clothing cannot be replaced, then it must be covered with a layer of non-breathing material, such as a plastic rain suit, to prevent evaporation. It is very important to also place an insulation layer over this rain suit to prevent the increased conduction of heat through the wet fabric from further allowing a rapid heat loss.

A rain suit cover could also act as a wind breaker to help contain convection heat loss. Its use in preventing evaporation over damp clothing during a rescue operation has merit only if additional insulation is placed over the rain suit. Its use over insulation that is dry may at times be detrimental due to the accumulation of moisture, thus decreasing the thermal efficiency of the underlying garments.

Increase heat production

The greatest increase of internal heat production occurs with volitional activity -- that is doing the work of walking, skiing, chopping wood, etc. If a person feels himself becoming cold, is relatively rested, has work to do or feels that they may exercise without undue loss of energy reserves, then volitional work is an excellent method of increasing the core temperature. Simply put: if you feel yourself getting chilly or starting to shiver, you may either put on more clothes, get out of the cold weather, or get active enough that you no longer feel cold. The increased heat production from volitional activities is indicated by Figure 10 (page 33), while heat production from shivering is discussed on page 32.

TREATMENT OF PROFOUND HYPOTHERMIA

If a member of your party is cold and exhausted, the method of having them walk or otherwise perform activities to heat themselves from the core out will not work. The exhausted person will have too little energy substrate reserve to allow this technique to work for long. It is mandatory in these cases to take every measure possible to prevent further heat loss in this individual. This person needs: protection from further heat loss; rest; nutrition so that their energy substrates can be replenished over the next several hours; and external heat if that is convenient.

Shivering and vasoconstriction are not indicators of impending hypothermia. These activities represent the body fine tuning its heat conservation and heat production. They do indicate a heat loss greater than your current activity is producing. Uncontrolled shivering IS an indicator of hypothermia, as opposed to mild shivering in response to cold air on the skin or the initial phases of mild hypothermia. If the person has limited energy stores and volitional work or shivering is not desirable, additional insulation must be acquired or other protection from the environment sought.

As mentioned elsewhere, it is difficult to assess the state of hypothermia from symptoms. The symptoms of deepening hypothermia noted in Figure 1 (page 4), include indicators of profound hypothermia. The person who is obtunded, unable to shiver, who is very clumsy -- this individual is dangerously hypothermic. This person will need help in order to survive.

Helping the profoundly hypothermic victim to survive in the field is not an easy task. Frequently, the circumstances are such that both rescuer and victim are in severe weather circumstances and both may be in danger. In helping the severely hypothermic, or the person at risk in becoming severely hypothermic (such as a person who fell into cold water or a person with the symptoms of early hypothermia who is exhausted), it is essential that further heat loss be prevented. Wet clothing must be handled as mentioned above.

As indicated elsewhere the use of hot liquids and the stuffing of candy or other nutrients into the victim will do little immediate good. The ideal would be to get the victim into a warm environment. Warm liquids by mouth, even breathing heated air, might cause a reflex vasodilation in some people. This is possibly more of a theoretical problem than a real one. Certainly if the victim is in a warm environment any vasodilation which occurs will do no harm (see the discussion on afterdrop, page 69). The warm water given will help with the important problem of dehydration; nutrients will eventually provide the source of energy; rest will allow the by-products of energy production to be cleansed from the muscle tissues and new high energy substrates to be formed from the nutrients that have been consumed.

Frequently the best shelter for a severely hypothermic victim available in the field will be a sleeping bag. If the victim is wet and can be transported as a litter case, his wet clothes should be removed and he should be placed in a sleeping bag for transport. If his clothes cannot be removed, then they should be covered with a waterproof cover, such as a rain suit, and the victim placed in the sleeping bag for transport. He will generally continue to cool under these conditions if he is profoundly hypothermic. People with a core temperature under 90°F (32.2°C) have generally consumed most readily available energy substrate. They are unable to produce heat from muscle shiver or work contraction. Their basal metabolic rate has been slowed and they will produce very little heat to combat the simple equilibration of cold from the extremities. They will experience an afterdrop not related to peripheral vasodilation -- it will amount to the leaching of heat from their core slowly into the cooled extremities by conduction through body tissues. They must be handled gently to avoid agitating their very irritable hearts. The slightest jar can cause a deadly ventricular fibrillation which will effectively stop their circulation and lead to a total cardiac standstill.

In the field with a very hypothermic victim, one who is probably below 90°F (32.2°C), when evacuation is not feasible, a method of rewarming as well as protecting from further heat loss must be undertaken.

On expeditions into the far north during winter conditions I take the precaution of bringing semi-rectangular sleeping bags that twin. The warmest bag for weight is a mummy bag as there is minimal extra space to heat. A semi-rectangular bag has more weight and inside space which must be heated by the occupant. But it also provides room in which to maneuver into and out of clothes. When it's 40° below zero, and there is no heat for the tent, dressing and undressing inside a sleeping bag prevents considerable heat loss. It also provides the best method of hypothermia rescue available under sub-zero and remote conditions.

With the sleeping bags twinned it is feasible to place the victim inside and have the rescuer crawl in, undressing both the victim and himself with minimal further exposure to the cold. This process takes some time. Considerable energy is consumed and heat developed by this activity. A twinned bag is large enough, that once the victim and rescuer are naked, a second rescuer may enter and similarly undress. The second rescuer is a valuable help as this additional thermal mass will greatly aid the rewarming process with greater safety and less energy drain for the rescuers.

Rescuer(s) and victim should huddle together. Hat, scarf, or other clothing should be lightly wrapped around the face or used to plug the entrance of the bag to help capture warm breath and prevent the breathing of cold air. Straddling the trunk will not waste valuable heat on the extremities, which are vasoconstricted and which will slowly rewarm inside the bag anyway. It is probable that afterdrop will not occur due to this extremity rewarming process, but will actually be decreased due to the additional heat being provided by the rescuer(s). Without this outside source of heat, the hypothermic victim with a profound core temperature depression may simply continue the cooling process due to a lack of adequate metabolic substrate.

An early recorded testimony to the value of cuddling a hypothermic victim dates back to an early journal of Arctic exploration. Dr. Richardson, a physician on the Sir John Franklin Expedition to the Hood River in Arctic Canada in 1821, directed the rescue of a party member who had capsized in an icy rapids. The account reads:

> "Belanger was suffering extremely, immersed to his middle in the center of the rapid, the temperature of which was very little above the freezing point, the upper part of his body covered with wet clothes, exposed in a temperature not much above zero, to a strong breeze.... By direction of Dr. Richardson, he was instantly stripped, and being rolled up in blankets, two men undressed themselves and went to bed with him; but it was some hours before he recovered his warmth and sensations."
> — From Narrative of a Journey to the Shores of the Polar Sea in the Years 1819, 20, 21 by Sir John Franklin

When in doubt about how hypothermic a person may be, treat as if they were profoundly hypothermic. Treat very gently; prevent further heat loss; arrange evacuation; provide rewarming in a slow, controlled manner such as indicated above. Attached as Appendix I are official State of Alaska, Division of Public Health, Emergency Medical Services Section, protocols for the treatment of both chronic and acute hypothermia by all levels of rescue personnel.

The naked cuddling of a hypothermia victim may be dangerous to the rescuer. A survey taken during the previous year of Search & Rescue organizations around the United States has reported 12 incidences of two huddled victims, naked and dead in a sleeping bag. What this statistic does not tell you is the condition of the rescuer, who may have also been hypothermic, and the condition of their sleeping bag which may have been wet or faulty to the degree that additional large amounts of heat were being lost to the environment. Prevention of heat loss via conduction to the cold ground is critical. What these statistics do not tell us is the number of people who may have been saved using this technique. Data such as this would seldom be reported by survivors who have extricated themselves.

MANAGING THE COLD HEART

It was noted that many victims of hypothermia were arriving in emergency rooms profoundly cold, but alive, only to die during the attempted rewarming. Postmortem examinations of hypothermic victims reveal a variety of pathological changes, but the exact cause of death has been a hotly debated subject.

The heart appears particularly vulnerable, with very slow heart rates developing as the core temperature lowers. Generally the heart rate may be expected to decrease 10 beats per minute for every degree Fahrenheit of core temperature drop. A change in the electrocardiogram called the "J" or Osborne wave may develop which is supposedly a specific electrocardiogram indicator of hypothermia, but many cases may be seen without this particular finding (see Figure 21). An irregular heart rate called atrial fibrillation is frequent in cold hearts. By itself this arrhythmia poses no threat to life.

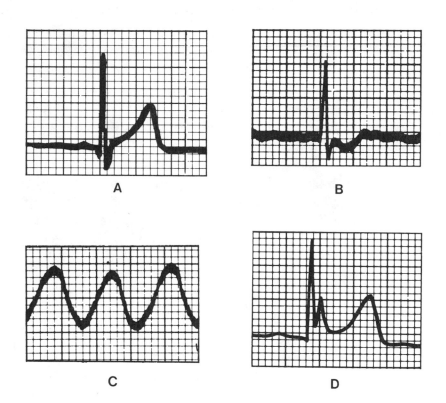

FIGURE 21   "ELECTROCARDIOGRAPH TRACINGS"

The above electrocardiograph (ECG or EKG) tracings are discussed in the text. A. Normal tracing. B. Atrial fibrillation. C. The very dangerous and pre-lethal ventricular fibrillation. D. The Osborne or "J" wave noted in some cases of hypothermia.

However, as core temperature drops the heart may suddenly go into ventricular fibrillation. This arrhythmia causes the heart to fail to provide any effective pumping action. Worse, ventricular fibrillation soon degenerates into a total heart standstill or asystole -- cardiac death.

While it is known that cold predisposes the heart to ventricular fibrillation, there are many events which initiate it. The slightest jar is enough to produce such a lethal event in the cold heart. For this reason gentle handling of all hypothermia victims is mandatory. There is concern that tickling the throat will produce ventricular fibrillation through a pharyngeal reflex. Some authorities have warned that drinking hot liquid would possibly be enough to produce it. Certainly CPR would cause a profound chance of ventricular fibrillation and for that reason, once initiated CPR must be continued until the victim is shown to have a functioning, regular pulse rate or acceptable electrocardiogram tracing.

If a known hypothermic is found, unconscious, with no detectable heart rate, and the victim can be transported -- it is best to protect from further heat loss and transport gently. The application of CPR in this case is being studied at the present moment. It has been shown that CPR in hypothermic dogs fails to move blood, probably due to its viscosity. It is obvious that CPR is a type of rough handling that we generally try to avoid when dealing with hypothermic victims. The normal methods of electric countershock to start a heart will not work in cold hearts -- those with a core temperature below 85°F (30°C). A cold heart must be warmed to above that temperature to start it with DC countershock. If CPR has been started, it is mandatory that it be continued until the victim has reached a treatment facility and warmed to the point that DC countershock can be given and the heart restarted.

The technique for the application of cardio-pulmonary resuscitation, and in fact its very use in hypothermia, are matters of current research and interest in the scientific community. It is well established that the cold heart is a delicate object -- rough handling of the victim, even by bouncing the victim on a litter, can cause the heart to develop the lethal erratic beat known as ventricular fibrillation which can lead to total heart stoppage, or asystole. It is primarily the concern that the aggressive chest compressions encountered during CPR may cause ventricular fibrillation and asystole that causes the controversy over the use of CPR on the cold heart.

On one hand there are several factors that indicate that CPR might be best for a hypothermic victim:

1. CPR causes a change in thoracic pressure and does not actually squeeze the heart, so that properly done the heart should not be traumatized.

2. Cold blood does not give up its oxygen as readily to tissue as warm blood, thus it is important to insure adequate blood flow.

3. Cold blood is very thick or viscous, and its movement by a very slow heart beat should be augmented by CPR.

4. The cold victim may have had a heart attack requiring CPR to aid in his recovery during the warming process.

5. It has been difficult to teach our population to start CPR on the person with no heart beat, changing the rules might confuse people with minimal exposure to CPR training.

On the other hand there are several reasons for modifying the use of CPR in the hypothermic victim.

1. No matter how gentle and proper the technique, the possibility of inducing a fatal arrythmia is present.

2. Since the metabolic rate has been slowed considerably, there is much less need for oxygen by body tissues and a very slow or undetectable heart rate may be tolerated.

3. It is possible that a cold heart which is not beating, may not be able to respond to the intrathoracic pressure changes of CPR to cause any blood movement regardless of how proper the technique has been applied.

4. A slow beating heart, which may not be detectable to rescuers, may be providing enough perfusion of tissue to prevent cell death.

Attempting to increase this rate of perfusion may be adding additional risk without help.

Currently, several paramedic protocols in this country do not have CPR started in a "known hypothermic," but rather have the victim transported to a medical facility where he is simply monitored until the body is warmed adequately for countershock. This is not universally accepted, but it is probably the best approach. It will be several years before current research in this area provides the answers.

Attached as Appendix I is the protocol suggested by the State of Alaska for hypothermia and cold water near drowning. This protocol requires the use of CPR, although it is my understanding that certain local protocols do not have paramedic personnel start CPR in a "known hypothermic" who does not have evidence of cardiac activity.

"AFTERDROP" -- ITS SIGNIFICANCE

It was also noted that the rewarming of the cold victim seemed to cause a paradoxical further lowering of the core temperature, called "afterdrop." As indicated in Figure 22, the victim's core temperature took a further downward plunge once external heat was applied. It has been feared that "afterdrop" could initiate the dreaded ventricular fibrillation and be a primary cause for the death of the rescued victim.

An "afterdrop" curve (see next page), demonstrates a continued decrease in the victim's core temperature after the rewarming process has been started. At first this was thought to be due to vasodilation and thus made more profound by rapid rewarming.

The mechanism for "afterdrop" was felt to be related to the sudden vasodilation or opening of the peripheral blood vessels, thus dumping cold blood into the core. It has subsequently been found, however, that even inanimate objects such as watermelons and dead

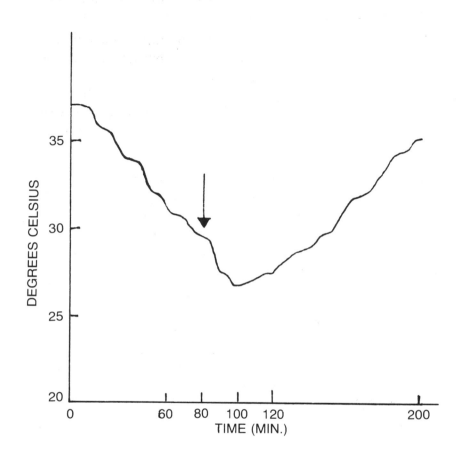

FIGURE 22   "AFTERDROP"
The arrow indicated the point at which heat has been applied to the subject. Rather than an instant warming trend, a continued cooling is noted. This has been termed "afterdrop" and is discussed in the text.

pigs have afterdrop when being heated again. Vasodilation is obviously not the cause of afterdrop.

   If an object, such as a watermelon (which is much more pleasant to work with than a dead pig) starts out at a nice warm temperature and is placed in freezing water, the core temperature will remain at the same level for a period of time. As the heat is removed by the cold water, the core temperature will begin to drop. The exterior of the melon might be quite cold, but the center is slowly equilibrating, losing its heat to the cold surroundings. A temperature gradient will exist from a cold exterior to a still warmer interior. Now if this melon is placed in very warm water, the core temperature will continue to drop before the warmth causes a temperature rise. The degree of this afterdrop in the melon seems to be directly related to the rapidity of cooling. If the melon is placed in water that is cool, but not at the freezing point, its afterdrop will be less profound. If the cooling melon is placed in very warm water, the afterdrop does not become more pronounced, than if it were placed in lukewarm water.

Afterdrop was blamed for many of the deaths associated with the rewarming process. It was imagined that this continued cooling was responsible for fatal cardiac arrhythmias. If vasodilation was the method by which afterdrop occured, then a rapid rewarming technique would be counter-indicated as it would cause a more profound afterdrop from the larger amount of cold blood suddenly returning to the core from the cold surface skin.

Current research has indicated that afterdrop is not due to vasodilation from rapid reheating, that it is not the cause of increased mortality when using rapid reheating techniques, that the amount of afterdrop is dependent upon the rate of cooling that is occurring, and that increased mortality in the very hypothermic victim is from loss of the metabolic control as discussed on page 45.

SUDDEN HYPOTHERMIA DURING INTENSIVE EXERCISE IN WINTER ATHLETES

It is not an uncommon event to hear of an athlete during a winter competition in x-country skiing suddenly collapsing of hypothermia. Frequently the person was noted to be sweating pro-fusely by fellow competitors just prior to the collapse. Their clothes have been noted to be wet with sweat, yet they have been profoundly cold when reached shortly after their collapse. How could a person who must have been overheating become hypothermic so suddenly?

There is no experimental evidence to tell us precisely what has occurred, but I surmise that the following explains the development of their distress. I doubt that these people have been hypothermic very long. Their heat loss has been accelerated due to profuse sweating from an initial overheating problem. The high energy output they are producing during the competition allows them to remain in a sort of thermal balance until their energy substrate becomes decreased to the point that they are no longer able to maintain the same level of work and heat generation. A high heat loss level is caused by the wet clothing, hair, and skin as well as vasodilation. A rapid fall in body temperature ensues. The athlete in complete exhaustion is probably suffering from dehydration due to the sweating and rapid breathing. This further jeopardizes the thermal control. Collapsing on the ground will increase conduction heat loss adding to the rapid convection losses mentioned. The athlete rapidly becomes hypothermic.

It turns out that long hair is not an advantage during winter. Heat loss studies of the human head have been performed by Dr. Richard Pozos of the University of Minnesota School of Medicine at Duluth where it was found that a long haired head offered no additional protection over a bald head. The insulating property of human hair is not a significant factor. Wet hair from physical activity might make it more of a detriment than a sweaty, but easily dried, bald head.

Field Management of Acute Hypothermia

Cold Water Immersion and Submersion

Falling into cold water will rapidly induce hypothermia. This "acute" or "immersion" hypothermia has many different characteristics from the slowly developing "chronic" hypothermia of cold weather exposure. The body can bring some special protective reflexes into play, but there are also some dangerous reflexes that may occur. Survival is modified by the water and air temperature, protective clothing and physical condition of the victim, types of physiological responses of the victim, immersion or submersion of the victim, evidence of near drowning, and resources of the rescuers.

Water temperature plays a major role in the length of survival. If water temperature is above 68°F (20°C), hypothermia should not result. However, most people will die of hypothermia within 6 hours if the water temperature is lower than 59°F (15°C) and within 1 hour in water temperature at the freezing point.

There are three primary ways in which death can occur during cold water immersion. As cold water will conduct heat at a rate 20 times that of air at the same temperature, the most common problem will be a continual cooling resulting in possible confusion at a core temperature of about 95°F (35°C) and unconsciousness at roughly 90°F (32°C) with subsequent drowning. Others may abruptly drown from the reflex involuntary gasping of ice water immersion. More

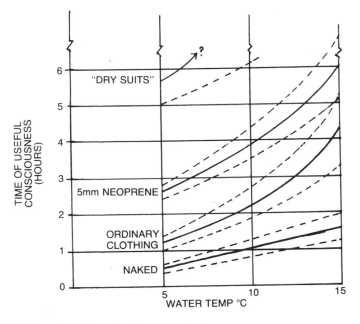

FIGURE 23 "COLD WATER SURVIVAL"

The above graph demonstrates the time of useful consciousness in hours for various water temperatures and conditions of dress.

rarely the sudden shock of ice water entry may cause immediate cardiac death from ventricular fibrillation. If a proper personal flotation device (life jacket or PFD) is being worn, the victim's head should be kept out of the water. It is then possible for them to cool into unconsciousness without drowning.

Hypothermia can protect a person in whom cardiac arrest has occurred, as mentioned elsewhere. But acute immersion hypothermic victims who have had cardiac arrest have a much poorer chance of survival than those who have not. When rescuing an immersion hypothermic victim it is very important to prevent any rough handling as the heart will be very sensitive and ventricular fibrillation may be accidentally induced. This is true of the victim who is walking, talking, and in every way seems to be behaving normally. After cold water immersion this victim must be made to lay down and treated as a litter case. Vasoconstriction will have allowed their skin temperature to have cooled as low as the water temperature, while the core temperature may be quite high, even above 95°F (35°C). Equilibration of this temperature will result in a core cooling.

If the victim is moving on their own, blood flow will cause a considerable afterdrop which may well precipitate a lethal cardiac arrhythmia. The ideal treatment for such a victim is immediate hot water 110°F (43.3°C) immersion. This is the technique employed primarily in England where they have had extensive experience with acute immersion hypothermia from North Sea disasters during war time and most recently due to oil drilling platform accidents. The use of hot water immersion has been the subject of considerable debate. There are those who are concerned that a sudden vasodilation would occur causing a severe afterdrop. But the British experience has been that people do better with the hot water immersion technique. It is likely that the very cold extremities of these people will cause a considerable afterdrop via equilibration of this cold mantle with the available heat in the core. Hot water immersion may rapidly warm this skin layer and cause less of an afterdrop during the heat equilibration process.

The importance of treating people who appear so normal that they are able to walk, carry on conversations, and in all respects act as if they are not injured has been made repeatedly. In 1980 sixteen Danish fishermen were forced to jump into the North Sea when their fishing boat floundered. They were in the water for about 1½ hours before another boat was able to reach them. It lowered a cargo net to them. These men were still capable of climbing aboard via the net. They crossed the deck on their own and went below to the galley where they were supposed to have hot drinks and warm up. Instead, each one of these men died from hypothermia.

In the field, tubs of hot water will probably not be available, unless a cabin or other facility is near by. After immersion in water below 45°F (7.2°C), the breathing survivor should be stripped naked and placed in a sleeping bag with one, or preferably two, naked rescuers. The victim may not feel the necessity of such careful treatment, but careful rewarming with an outside heat source is best. If only a mummy style sleeping bag is available, dry the victim and place him in the bag. He may be given warm liquids by mouth, but expect a core temperaure afterdrop due to the tremendous amount of cold in the mantle which must equilibrate with the warmer core. Clothes may be warmed and placed in the bag with the victim. Care should be taken with objects that might lie against the person and cause thermal burns on the numb and delicate skin.

Cliff Jacobson in his book *CANOEING WILD RIVERS* (ICS Books, 1984) relates a tragic death of a famous and highly experienced expedition canoeist in 1955 on the Dubawnt River in the Northwest Territories:

"The sad irony is that Arthur Moffat might have survived his dunking on the Dubawnt River had his crew understood the nature of hypothermia. Evidently Moffat's friends believed his authoritative cries of 'I'm okay, I'm okay,' and simply placed him in a sleeping bag inside his tent. There was no 'sandwich treatment' or hot drink."

If the person has experienced cold water immersion and the air temperature is subzero, it will frequently be impossible to remove the frozen clothes. When alone the victim may roll in snow which will freeze to the outer clothing and form an icy shell which will provide some wind and thermal protection. This is a desperate situation and building a fire may be the only chance for survival. On several occasions I have had members of my party, myself included, fall through ice in freezing temperatures. We never rolled in snow, but each time our clothes rapidly froze. Fortunately we were able to get a fire started and totally warm and dry ourselves. Once, two members of my expedition beat a hasty retreat in their frozen clothes to the cabin they had just left. They were able to make a fire in the stove rapidly as they had prepared a fire lay prior to their departure. This rapid movement can be lethal as was mentioned in the case of the Danish fishermen. But when there are no other choices, obtaining warmth must be rapidly attempted before the numbing effect of the cold makes action impossible. Cold water immersion in subfreezing, and certainly in subzero, temperatures is a desperate situation. I think everyone recognizes this. What people do not recognize is the danger cold water immersion has even when the air temperature is above freezing.

Cold water SUBMERSION[1] is always associated with asphyxiation and simultaneous hypothermia. The asphyxiation results in rapid brain death so the prompt rescue and immediate implementation of CPR play an important role in the survival of the victim. Total submersion in cold water results in rapid core cooling which results in a lower oxygen demand by the brain and other body tissues and increases the chance of survival over that of a victim of warm water submersion. These rapid cooling rates in very cold water submersion result from the normal conduction and convection losses of heat as experienced by the cold water immersion victim, and in addition increased losses from the submerged head with its large unprotected blood flow and to a less extent from core cooling due to cold water swallowing and pulmonary aspiration.

[1] There is a distinct difference between immersion and submersion. Submersion indicates that the victim is entirely under water; immersion means that the head is above water.

Children are cooled more rapidly than adults due to their larger surface area to volume ratio. They frequently have less subcutaneous fat for insulation than an adult. And in children up to the age of 2 or 3 there at times can exist a circulatory reflex called the "mammalian diving reflex." The immersion of the child's face triggers this reflex which causes oxygenated blood to move from the lungs to the heart and brain, the heart rate to slow to several beats per minute, and a shutting of the epiglottis which protects the lungs from water while submerged. Rapid cooling decreases the oxygen requirement and the brain is protected by the oxygen rich blood which has been shunted to it during the initial phase of this reflex. This reflex can extend the underwater survival for the children to slightly beyond 30 minutes.

Older persons resuscitated successfully are probably not beneficiaries of the mammalian diving reflex, but of the rapidly induced hypothermia of cold water submersion. Full recovery after 10 to 40 minutes of submersion can occur, even in adults. Because of this, CPR must be immediately started in all apparently drowned immersion and submersion hypothermia victims and continue aggressively. It is a law in Denmark that a cold water drowning victim can only be declared dead when they are warm and dead. If the victim remains unresponsive after being warmed to 86°F (30°C), they may be considered dead. It may take several hours of CPR while the victim is being properly rewarmed to make this determination. The hospital management of victims of cold water submersion is very complex. These victims are best transferred to centers with experience with this problem, but the victim will never have a chance if the rescuers do not implement CPR immediately. (See Appendix I.)

SELF PRESERVATION TECHNIQUES IN WATER

Death from submersion in water has been a serious aspect of man's dependency upon bodies of water for transportation, food, and recreation since the beginning of time. Today there are an estimated 140,000 deaths from drowning worldwide, yearly, with at least 8,000 of these occurring in the United States.

Knowing how to swim would be an apparent aid in preventing drowning, but statistically amongst those groups who know how to swim there is a higher risk of drowning. This probably represents more exposure to water and the engagement in activities that non-swimmers would avoid. I would regard knowing how to swim as mandatory for anyone planning on engaging in canoeing or other forms of water sport. It should be a skill learned by everyone.

Several years ago a new technique to allow long term survival in the water was developed called "drownproofing." This was a technique of flotation which minimized the movements made, thus conserving energy. It is a breath holding maneuver, using minimal kicking strokes to return the victim to the surface. On the surface, a sudden kick (even with the legs tied together) allows the person to raise their face to air and grab a quick breath. The action of blowing out air and raising the head normally causes the person to sink under water. As they have fully expanded lungs, they will soon float to the surface where the process is repeated. Drownproofing is a valuable personal skill which I have been able to teach to any of my boy scouts without difficulty.[1]

Unfortunately, the frequent submersion of the head required in using the drownproofing technique increases heat loss in cold water. It has been estimated that a person using drownproofing in 50°F (10°C) water will have an average survival time of 1½ hours. Treading and swimming in the same temperature water might extend survival to a little over 2 hours. Holding still in a personal flotation device (life jacket) could increase the survival time to almost 3 hours. A technique of assuming a curled up position in a life jacket, called the HELP *(heat escape lessening posture)* may extend survival time in the same temperature water to over 4 hours. A similar heat preserving technique has been designed for 2 or more people with life jackets in the water, the HUDDLE position. By placing the life jackets on backwards, persons can hug each other so that the chest, groin, and legs can be pressed together, thus preserving some of the body heat from the cold convection currents (see Figures 24 and 25).

[1] An excellent reference for this technique is *DROWNPROOFING* by Michael Bettsworth, Schocken Books, 200 Madison Avenue, New York City, NY 10016, $2.95.

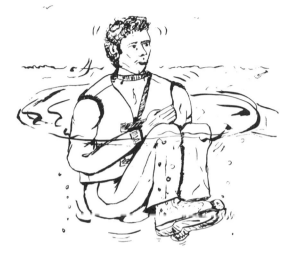

FIGURE 24   ''THE H.E.L.P. POSITION''
The Heat Escape Lessening Posture. By decreasing the body surface area and protecting the groin and abdomen, the victim can lessen heat loss if he does not roll in the water or go awash in waves.

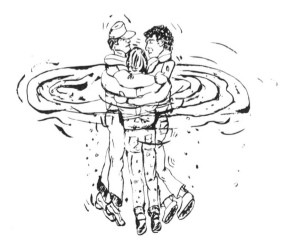

FIGURE 25   ''THE HUDDLE POSITION''
Heat loss can be decreased when members of a group huddle together, providing some convection loss protection. This technique helps keep the group together, but it is difficult to actually minimize heat loss in real life due to bobbing action and the different floating characteristics which many people have.

Several aspects of advocating the HELP and HUDDLE technique must be mentioned. While they seem theoretically beneficial, controlled experiments at the University of Minnesota Medical School at Duluth have failed to demonstrate the expected difference in core cooling rate of either HELP or HUDDLE. Dr. Pozos, a respected authority in hypothermia research, feels this is due to the technical difficulty of performing these maneuvers. He advises practicing the HELP position with the same life jacket that you might be using in the cold water. With many models and individual body builds, the person assuming the curled up position will roll in the water, allowing repeated cold water exposure to the head and back of the neck. This causes more of a heat loss through this area than one saves from decreasing the abdominal/groin heat loss. It would be unlikely that any practice before a cold water immersion could be expected to take place. If in assuming the HELP position you find yourself rolling around or awash with cold water, Dr. Pozos recommends simply crossing your legs at the ankles and bringing the thighs together. This should minimize heat loss, while not allowing you to roll around in the water. The HUDDLE position can prove very difficult as each member of the HUDDLE group needs to be balanced with regard to their flotation level and size. People tend to float at different levels, even with life jackets on. An unbalanced group constantly allows members to go awash and requires excessive struggling to keep in balance. Prior dunking practice with the same "HUDDLE group" is again impossible to achieve normally, but almost essential for this technique to adequately work. The best aspect of the HUDDLE method is that it keeps a group together for psychological benefit and possibly would be an aspect of improved ease in rescue.

A technique that has saved the lives of many people who have found themselves trapped aboard a sinking ship in cold waters has been for them to put on as many layers of clothing they could find. If possible, the outer layer should be covered with a rain suit to decrease the effects of conduction currents. A large life jacket then covers the rain suit. Having the foresight to take these simple measures, if time permits, can extend your cold water survival time considerably.

Many advocates of the HELP and HUDDLE positions have degraded the drownproofing method of emergency flotation, due to its increased heat loss in cold water. While this system will cause a decreased survival time in cold water of 50°F (10°C) or cooler, as a method of survival in water -- particularly without a life jacket -- it is a valuable skill that should be taught and learned.

Alcohol -- Its Role in Hypothermia and Other Cold Related Injuries

Alcohol is a powerful vasodilator. Doses as little as 1 ounce of 80 proof alcohol will cause the blood vessels to open. Under the conditions of cold stress, the vasoconstriction of blood vessels is an essential and early step in the preservation of core heat. By causing vasodilation and decreased insulation, a rapid heat loss could result from alcohol use in a cold environment.

The warm flush one feels when drinking alcohol is evidence of vasodilation. It represents a surge of warmer blood from the core being released to the surface over the dilated blood vessel system. This comfort is not dangerous as long as the core temperature is not depressed, for not only is the surface being warmed but the core is simultaneously being cooled. While it is permissible for chilly skiers to enjoy hot toddys around a fireplace in a ski lodge, it would be a mistake to enjoy the warm flush of alcohol if there was any chance of being exposed further to cold temperatures. The use of the alcohol would have lowered the core temperature some-what already and would have further blocked the important vas-oconstriction protective mechanism for preventing further body heat loss.

A further problem with the use of alcohol when traveling in wilderness situations is the obvious effect which it has on mental function. This reason certainly outweighs even the dangers of hypothermia as a significant problem. The loss of mental function, or even the slight blunting of reflexes and intelligent decision making abilities, can easily result in disaster -- and all too frequently has.

At autopsy there have been a large number of cases of young and otherwise healthy people who have died of hypothermia with blood alcohol levels of 150 to 300 mg per deciliter. While this level represents intoxication, it is not great enough to have caused loss of mental function to the point that the victim should have been unaware of danger. Further, while vasodilation will cause some heat loss, laboratory studies in humans and lab animals fail to show substantial heat loss through the skin. Studies have shown an apparent downward setting of the brain's thermostat (hypothalamus) which impairs heat production. At an alcohol level of only moderate intoxication (150 mg per deciliter) this deactivation can lead to a rapid fall in core temperature at ambient temperatures of 39.2°F (4°C) which could prove rapidly fatal.

The use of alcohol in the outdoors must be generally condemned. The fact that it is used frequently must be recognized, and its potential deleterious effects on the hypothermic victim anticipated. Additional insulation for a person who has consumed alcohol is essential. A person does not have to be drunk to require this special protection from hypothermia.

Conversely we might ask, does alcohol protect from death by hypothermia? Hypothermia induced death frequently occurs when core temperature has reached the 79°F (26°C) range. Yet, in a search of the literature at least 35 cases of survival of core temperatures of 77°F (25°C) or lower have occurred in persons heavily intoxicated with alcohol, barbiturates, or other metabolic suppression agents.

A particular effect of these agents is the depression or elimination of the shiver response to a dropping core temperature. Another frequently is vasodilation which would cause a more rapid heat loss and a quick onset of profound hypothermia. As the energy substrate muscle glycogen was not consumed by the cooling victim, perhaps this meant that there was more energy available for internal rewarming. Perhaps the more rapid onset approached that of the acute or immersion hypothermic victim without the profound metabolic changes that accompany gradual or chronic hypothermia.

In small laboratory animals it has been noted that alcohol reduced the frequency of ventricular fibrillations, cardiac arrest, the mean lethal temperature, and the temperature of restarting the heart in hypothermic subjects.

What the above does not take into account, is the number of alcoholic victims of hypothermia that do not make it. These deaths probably outweigh the numbers of alcoholic survivors of hypothermia by a large ratio, but the statistics would be very hard to gather. Frequently the cause of death will not be listed as hypothermia. Obviously, however, more research is required on first the normal response to hypothermia and then the protective mechanisms that may or may not exist from alcohol or other suppressor substances.

A cold stress related injury where alcohol CAN play a therapeutic role is in the treatment of immersion, or trench, foot (see "immersion foot," page 111).

Diurnal Temperature Variation

A Possible Danger to Cave Explorers and Winter Arctic Travelers

A possible risk for the induction of hypothermia may exist for cave explorers, arctic travelers, and others who remove themselves from a normal day-night pattern of living.

John Hunter, the English anatomist, discovered in 1778 that the body core temperature varies during the day according to a 24 hour cycle, or circadian rhythm. Many physiological and psychological patterns follow this circadian rhythm which has been proven to be controlled within the organism, probably by a portion of the brain called the hypothalamus. Within that structure are two sections that synchronize these built in cycles. One section controls a natural sleep-wake cycle and changes in plasma levels of various hormones such as growth hormone, urinary calcium excretion, etc. The other section controls body core temperature rhythm and changes in other hormones such as plasma cortisol levels and rapid eye movement (REM) during sleep.

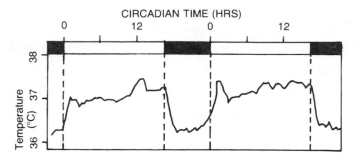

FIGURE 26   "CIRCADIAN RHYTHM - TEMPERATURE/DAY-NIGHT CYCLE"
In humans there is a 1.8°F (1°C) temperature difference between the normal core temperature during the day and at night.

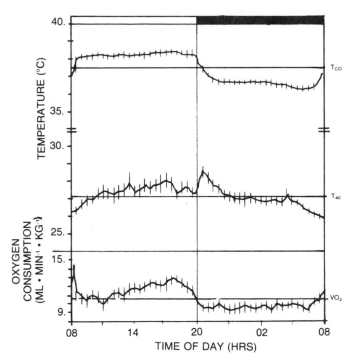

FIGURE 27   "SKIN HEAT LOSS AND HEAT PRODUCTION DURING THE
                 CIRCADIAN CYCLE"
Core temperature is displayed in the upper panel. Skin temperature in the middle panel is an indicator of heat loss. Its initial high level during the first part of the night (black bar) coupled with the decrease in basal metabolic heat output, shown from oxygen consumption values in the bottom panel, causes the rapid drop in core temperature characteristic of the circadian rhythm. (Adapted from Moore-Ede in Pozos and Wittmers *The Nature and Treatment of Hypothermia*, University of Minnesota Press, 1983)

When men are placed in conditions where they lose contact with the day-night cycle, these circadian rhythms continue to follow closely to, but are significantly different from the 24 hour cycle. The endogenous controls of body temperature rhythm and sleep-wake cycles are synchronized by contact with the normal day-night exposure, or through artificially timing food intake patterns to match appropriate points in the day-night cycle. If removed for extended periods from normal day-night contact, the cycles become desynchronized with the body temperature cycle not matching the sleep-wake cycle.

Figure 27 demonstrates the relationship of core heat production and skin heat loss with the day-night cycle. Core heat production drops during the early night as seen from the drop in oxygen consumption, while an increase in vasodilation causes increased skin temperature allowing heat loss and accelerating the core temperature drop in the early evening. This is followed by a skin temperature drop which shows a heat conservation that helps maintain the core temperature from further drop. With daylight, the diurnal skin temperature change at rest allows skin temperature increase to match the increased core heat production, thus stabilizing core heat at slightly higher daytime baseline levels. Heat loss and heat production are then synchronized.

This daily change in the body's core temperature at rest may play an important role in the development of hypothermia in cave explorers and others, such as patients in an intensive care unit, where confusion of the brain's 24 hour clock cycle may occur. This temperature variation is dependent not only on diurnal variations in basal metabolic heat output, but also diurnal changes in control of heat loss. It has been shown that these functions are separately controlled. While the normal diurnal core temperature variation is only 1.8°F (1°C), if the functions of diurnal control of heat production become uncoupled with the control of heat loss, profound drops in core temperature are possible.

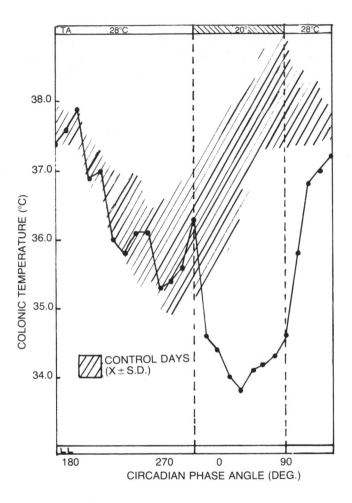

FIGURE 28   "CORE TEMPERATURE DROP DUE TO DESYNCHRONIZATION
WITH THE CIRCADIAN CYCLE"
The usual 1.8°F (1°C) drop during the circadian night cycle has been magnified during mild cold
stress in an animal confused with regard to its normal day-night cycle as described in the text.
(Adapted from Moore-Ede in Pozos and Wittmers *The Nature and Treatment of Hypothermia*,
University of Minnesota Press, 1983)

In Figure 28 the shaded area represents control values for a
24 hour circadian temperature cycle in a squirrel monkey whose
cycles have been desynchronized. Under a steady ambient temper-

ature of 82.4°F (28°C) a rectal temperature range is noted that varies from about 100°F (37.8°C) to 96.8°F (36°C). When the ambient temperature is dropped from 82.4°F (28°C) to 68°F (20°C), the core temperature is maintained in a normal circadian cycle with an appropriate rise, even in the presence of this mild cold stress. With the basal heat production cycle desynchronized from the heat conservation cycle, the result is instead a profound drop in core temperature to 93°F (33.9°C)!

Cave explorers, miners working day shifts, travelers in the winter Arctic regions could all become desynchronized unless attention is directed to a 24 hour life cycle based on meals, and sleep-awake cycles established by the clock. As seen above, the desynchronization of the basic circadian rhythms could allow the inducement of clinical hypothermia. For long underground expeditions, cave explorers (spelunkers) not only have to contend with frequently wet clothing and cool temperatures, but may have to avoid straying from an appropriate 24 hour circadian cycle.

6.   PROTECTION FROM THE COLD
Clothing Insulation -- The "Clo"

Insulation value of a garment is measured in a unit called a "clo." This is a thermal resistance unit and represents the property of a material to prevent the flow of heat from a warm body to a cold environment.

All of us have received outdoor clothing catalogs and have noted that sleeping bags and garments are frequently rated with a comfort range. It may indicate that a particular bag is good to 20°F (-6°C), 0°F (-17.7°C), or so forth. But when using this item in the field we may find that we have a difference of opinion! This is not the label maker's fault, but it reflects an inherent difference in people. Some people simply sleep warmer than others. Factors involved are the basal metabolic rate, amount of subcutaneous fat for insulation, psychological attitude, body surface area, and many minor determinants.

Wouldn't it be ideal to have a full-proof rating system? One that manufacturers, advertisers, and consumers could all agree upon? One so standardized that even federal regulations could be easily written with regard to an article's warmth rating?

Establishing a full-proof rating system could prevent disappointments with a manufacturer's claim for the warmth of a sleeping bag or garment. More importantly, it could provide the basis of wisely planning equipment for general or expedition use, without finding oneself dangerously under-equipped. The prevention of hypothermia is based upon insuring adequate protection.

Any such method would be best based on rating all garments by an actual insulation, or thermal resistance, unit. The building construction trade measures insulation using the term "R Factor." As mentioned above, the method designed for clothing is termed the "clo." These terms are convertible. In fact, to change an R Factor value to a clo multiply the R Factor by 1.136. To go the other direction, the clo would have to be multiplied by .88 to obtain the equivalent R Factor.

Clo units are interconvertible for metric or English measurement systems. Appendix II provides a formal definition of the clo unit and describes the terms for both metric and English measurement systems.

The total insulation of garments is additive. If the clo value of various articles is known, by adding these values together the total insulation provided by the ensemble can be computed. The value of 1 clo is approximately the insulation provided by a normal business suit, although the actual thermal resistance of the value can be quantitated mathematically.

Even a standardized system such as the clo does not directly indicate a comfort range, rather it precisely indicates the amount of resistance to nonevaporative heat loss per unit of surface area to provide a comfortable skin temperature of 89.6°F (32°C). With experience consumers would soon realize precisely what clo rating they would personally require to be comfortable under various temperature conditions while engaged in different activities. Figure 29 indicates the control of nonevaporative heat loss at different levels of activity and ambient temperatures.

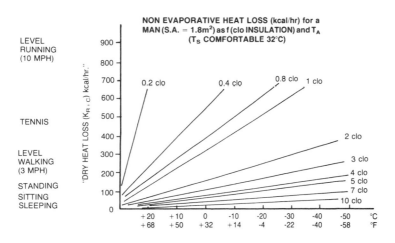

FIGURE 29   "HEAT LOSS VS. 'CLO' FACTOR AT A COMFORTABLE SKIN TEMPERATURE"

The use of different insulation amounts, expressed in clo factors, that would allow non-evaporative heat loss in kcal/hour for a standard sized man at different temperature ranges and activity levels to keep his skin a constant warm temperature (89.6°F or 32°C).

From the above graph it can be seen that a person at rest, generating 108 kcal per hour of metabolic heat, will require about 1 clo unit of insulation to be in thermal balance at 68°F (20°C). If the temperature were to drop to 32°F (0°C), he would require approximately 2.3 clo, and with a further temperature drop to -4°F (-20°C) his requirement would be 4.3 clo. An active skier generating 290 kcal of heat production due to his activity level even at a much lower temperature of -25°F (-31.7°C) would only need clothing that provided an effective clo of 2.0.

The clo value of a garment is dependent upon the materials from which it was constructed and its design. Easily compressed insulation, such as down, will lose its effectiveness at pressure points such as the shoulders if a jacket hangs heavily upon the wearer. Compression of insulation in sleeping bags against the cold ground requires less compressible insulation on the underneath side, or more practically the use of insulated foam pads for additional protection. Thermography studies, using infrared detectors to measure heat loss, have shown that a particular test parka, under wind chill tests, constructed with no zipper had a clo value of 2.04. With a zipper the clo value dropped to 0.93! Even more amazing was that the addition of a protected zipper cover and insulation tube increased the clo value to 2.17. Sewn through seams particularly lower the clo value. Baffled construction avoids this problem, but adds thickness, weight, and expense to an item. A sewn through construction technique is perfectly fine for clothing with lower clo value requirements, such as lightweight jackets, vests, etc.

Clothing Construction, Materials and Technique

A vacuum has the greatest insulation value of any material (or rather lack of it) known. There will be no conduction or convection loss of heat through a vacuum. Radiation loss will still occur, but it is curtailed by reflective insulation around the vacuum, the principle of the thermos bottle.

For practical purposes, the best insulation we can obtain for clothing and sleeping gear is dry, still air. The warmed layer of air which surrounds a human has a clo value of .78! Convection currents, of course, easily strip this insulation layer away. Insulation materials, such as down, Thinsulate, etc., will provide increased insulation because they stagnate or hold a thicker layer of air around the wearer. The less movement in this air, the better, for there is less heat loss via conduction currents.

Man's ability to leave a tropical climate to explore and populate the world was dependent upon his developing protection from the hostile environment, and this he primarily accomplished with clothes. The use of animal skins, tanned with wood smoke and rubbing techniques, provided a breathable, water resistant, wind proof insulation that, combined with various garment construction techniques, protected primitive man. For centuries fabrics constructed from natural plant fibers and from animal hair, feathers, or fur augmented hides as a construction material. The development of synthetic fibers such as nylon has had major technical and economic impact in clothing, tent, and sleeping bag construction for the outdoor traveler. Within the past few years improvements in these synthetic fibers have greatly increased our ability to protect ourselves.

A single sheet of cloth has a certain amount of insulating ability, depending upon the fibers from which it is constructed. Advances in fiber, insulation material as fill between sheets of fabric, and garment design are essential ingredients in optimizing our chances of comfort and even survival in the outdoors.

FIBER AND FABRIC CONSTRUCTION

Cotton has been a mainstay of fabric construction since ancient times. Its use in outdoor clothing cannot be condemned too highly. Designer and traditional brands of jeans have no place in the outdoors. Cotton allows heat to be conducted through it, even when dry, at a rate three times faster than wool, nylon, polyester, and acrylic fiber cloth. The latter four fibers are about equal in their dry insulation ability. Olefin (polypropylene) has about twice the dry insulation ability of those fibers and six times that of cotton. All manufacturers of outdoor clothing generally avoid pure cotton due to its poor insulation ability. Other major problems with cotton are its low evaporative ability and its very poor insulation ability when wet. Wet cotton allows thermal conductance to increase by a factor of 9 times, thus making it a danger to its wearer.

The use of 65 percent dacron with 35 percent cotton, however, provides strength, low cost, and rapid drying ability that makes this cloth, generally called 65-35 cloth, a good material for work clothes and for general outdoor wear. This is generally the material one finds when purchasing work clothes at major chain retail stores. I have used it on my canoe trips with total satisfaction. This cloth will actually dry itself after total immersion while being worn within one half hour on a day if the temperature is above 70°F (21°C) and the wearer is paddling a canoe or hiking at moderate rate. I wear this same garment over polypropylene underwear during winter travels.

Wool has been a mainstay of outdoor protection for years. It can be woven quite thick and with a tight weave for optimal insulation ability. It has the ability to suspend water vapor within its fibers while retaining its insulating ability. Wool garments have a low wicking ability which means that they are relatively difficult to dry, yet they feel relatively dry even when wet. Fabrics made from wool are very wear resistant, have moderate price, yet they are somewhat heavier than modern synthetics.

The synthetics nylon, polyester, and acrylic evaporate water readily, are close to wool in insulation ability, but they rapidly feel wet when damp. Nylon can be coated with different finishes to make excellent rain and wind proof garments or allowed to breath without coatings. It is very durable, relatively inexpensive and available in a variety of weights for different uses, from the heavy duty cloth of backpacks to light weight ripstop nylon cloth for sleeping bags and other breathable garments.

Olefin, or polypropylene, has been used as plastic sandwich bags for years. A recent innovation has been the production of a woven cloth from polypropylene fibers. Frequently called "polypro" this cloth has proven valuable in the construction of underwear -- either in net, lightweight weave, or heavy duty bulk weave. This cloth has great thermal insulation ability, almost twice that of wool. Measured as thermal conductance in kilocalories/square meter, polypro has a value of 1.2 compared to 2.1 for wool, 2.4 for nylon and most other synthetics, and the rather poor 6.1 of cotton.[1] This cloth has high wicking ability, to remove moisture from the skin and transfer it to outer garments. It evaporates rapidly and will not readily feel damp. Polypro underwear is a great advantage to active outdoors sports enthusiasts. This is particularly true of those activities requiring tremendous bursts of physical activity where a chance of sweating occurs, such as x-country ski racing.

Thermolactyl is a brand name for a cloth combining acrylic and polyester, used primarily as underwear. It combines the best characteristics of these two fabrics. People I have known who have used this product are very satisfied with it. Its cost is relatively high when compared to polypro.

Polyester pile garments are used for insulation as outer layers in spring/fall and middle layer insulation in winter clothing ensembles. As its fibers do not absorb water easily, these garments stay relatively dry and retain their insulation ability even if damp. These garments are fairly expensive. They wear well for several major trips, but even the best quality pile garments tend to become fuzzed and ragged after continual use and washings.

---

[1] Note the difference between thermal conductance vs. thermal resistance. These thermal conductance figures are a reflection of the ability of the substance to allow the conduction of heat. The larger the number the better the conductor and the poorer its insulation ability. The lower the number, the better its insulation ability.

The greatest natural insulation batting is eider down. Its high loft for its unit of weight results in considerable air trapping, the basis of clothing insulation, with very little garment weight. As it is highly compressible, bulky parkas and sleeping bags made with down will compress readily into small packages for ease in transportation when not in use. Frequently, pure down is augmented with a small percentage of feathers. This cuts the cost of the down mixture, but it also helps spring the down back into loft, once compression is removed. A major problem with down is the virtual total loss of insulation capability this substance has if it becomes wet. It is also expensive and in limited supply, most of it coming from mainland China.

Quallofil, PolarGuard, and Hollofil II are several synthetic fibers that have been developed especially for use as insulation batting. They perform far superior to cotton batting and to wool batting which has been used in the past. These fibers resist matting or clumping together, they drain water off when wet and still provide some thermal resistance when damp. These fibers have a high loft for their unit of weight. High loft fibers do not compress extremely well, but this can be an advantage also. Not compressing means that a person sleeping on a mat of these materials in a sleeping bag will not decrease their insulation capability with his body weight. They are less expensive than down or high grade feather mixtures.

Bulky garments produce less problems with the bellows effect, or drafts, due to their form fitting nature. If sewn with a quilting technique they lose considerable insulation capability for at the needle areas the fill is tightly compressed. This is eliminated with more costly sewing methods such as internal baffles, to prevent the loft from sliding from the top of a garment to the bottom, or by trapping the fill in tubes which can then be covered with inner and outer layers of cloth, or sewn as double layers of tubes.

Another recent development has been the production of microfilaments which produce very thin mats of insulation that still yield considerable insulation. Brand names in the United States of these products are 3M's Thinsulate, DuPont's Sontique, and Eastman

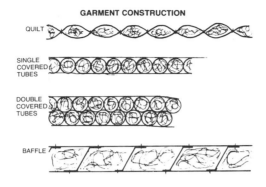

GARMENT CONSTRUCTION

FIGURE 30   "GARMENT CONSTRUCTION TECHNIQUES
The frequently found methods of garment and sleeping bag construction for cold weather use include the: A. Quilt or sewn through method; B. Single covered tubes; C. Double covered tubes; and D. Baffle construction.

Chemical's KodOlite. The filaments of Thinsulate and Sontique are 1/5th the diameter of Hollofil or PolarGuard, 4.5 microns in diameter compared to 25 microns. These microfilaments have about 2.1 times the insulation ability of an equal thickness of the older synthetic fiberfills. Their ability to provide such superior insulation with less thickness is due to superior air trapping by their small fibers. These fibers literally allow air to cling to them, just as the larger fibers do. But with more fibers per unit of volume, the amount of air trapped - and therefore the insulation or thermal resistance value - is greater. Like the larger fibers they do not retain water and will provide excellent insulation when wet. While they provide about twice the insulating value of the other fiberfills per unit of thickness, their denser structure means they weigh 30 to 40% as much per unit of thickness. Total weight of the newer material may end up being equal, with the newer material being only one half as thick. This increased density will not allow it to compress well into stuff sacks for carrying or storage. It is ideal in the construction of insulated gloves and other garments where bulk is a disadvantage.

Of the newer insulation materials mentioned above, Thinsulate is available in two varieties. Type B is 100% olefin and has little compression ability being primarily designed for footwear. Type C is 65% olefin and 35% polyester which is softer, more compressible and flexible for general garment use. Sontique is 100% polyester and very similar in characteristics to Thinsulate Type C. KodOlite is 100% polyester, but the fibers are a little larger, which places this insulation between the microfilaments and high-loft polyester insulations. It weighs about 15% more per unit of thickness and due to its larger fibers you will need more thickness to provide the same thermal resistance as the other two microfilaments.

BREATHABLE FABRICS vs VAPOR BARRIER

For centuries outdoors use has demonstrated the advisability of wearing breathable fabrics in cold weather. This allows the passage of water vapor from the skin to the outside atmosphere and minimizes the amount of water that would be absorbed by the wearer's clothing. As indicated, absorption of water vapor, or accidental wetting of garments, causes a loss of their insulating ability by decreasing their loft and allowing conduction heat loss and evaporative heat loss.

The problem with breathable outer fabrics is that they also leak water from rain, drizzle, and melting snow or sleet. This wetting from exterior atmospheric water sources can be minimized with the use of a water-proof outer covering. However, insensible moisture loss through the skin (page 30) as well as possible sweating can cause a considerable problem with moisture condensation on the interior surface of these waterproof outer covers. Frequently it pays not to wear an outer waterproof cover under conditions of light drizzle, as the amount of water that condenses on the inside of these jackets is considerably more than one would expect from the inclement weather.

It would seem that the ideal outer garment should be made from a material that would be wind proof, water repellent, and be water breathable. Several attempts were made to approach this ideal. Coatings have been developed for breathable cloths, such as canvas and cordura nylon, which would increase their water repellent nature while not decreasing their breathability. Special knitting techniques to provide this combination resulted in the production of Bulkflex and other materials. But the real breakthrough came with the introduction of a micro-pore filter, protected by lamination between breathable, wear resistant fabrics.

Water molecules coalesce into particles. The micro-pore layer would allow the passage of water vapor from the body as it is in small droplets of individual molecules to a few hundred molecules in size. This filter thus allows passage of vapor particles because its pores are about 700 times larger than a water molecule. Water from the atmosphere, even in its finest sprays, is a particulate clumping of hundreds of thousands of molecules which are not passed through the micropore membrane. It is essential, of course, that these delicate micro-pore membranes be protected with a laminate that breaths very well. The major micro-pore fabrics in use today are Gore-Tex, Stormshed, and Klimate. Extensive personal use with these fabrics have demonstrated that they work well, but that they do deteriorate with continual hard use. Considerable exposure to wood smoke accelerates this deterioration. Our parkas have been used on a daily basis for two years or more before failure, so the relative cost compared to the amount of use has been quite reasonable. These fabrics have been a valuable addition to the armamentarium of the outdoors traveler and investing in them is worth while for serious back country travelers or dwellers.

In the mid-1970s an aeronautical engineer, William Stephanson, popularized a new approach to outdoor wear, the vapor barrier system. This represented a 180 degree turn from the well proven breathable layer principle. Proponents of vapor barrier feel that it has two advantages. One is a decrease in dehydration and the other is the absolute protection of insulation from body moisture.

According to vapor barrier advocates the insensible moisture loss of the skin can be decreased by insuring a 100% layer of humidity on the surface. Insensible water loss is estimated to be about 1100 ml per day, divided between respiration and skin excretion. While sweating is an active process used by the body to control overheating, insensible skin moisture is a diffusion of moisture through interstitial cell spaces to outer skin layers. If this outer skin layer is dry, water continues to diffuse whereas if it is kept moist, the diffusion process literally stops.

Trying to determine if this system works as its advocates state is very difficult. A review of the physiology literature fails to provide much help. From personal experience, while camping for up to 13 days at temperatures at -20°F (-28.9°C) or below, the use of a vapor barrier liner in sleeping bags has been of tremendous help. Without the liners, the bags rapidly gain moisture, which freezes beneath the bag surface at what would have to be considered a "freeze layer." This freeze layer builds a mantle of ice that continues to trap all further water passed through the skin. It also provides insulation from the exterior bitter cold temperatures, even though the insulation value of the original sleeping bag material has been decreased considerably by this wetting process. Sleeping in these solidly frozen bags is not comfortable, but at that point one is generally worried about survival, not simple comfort. These bags become extremely heavy and if rolled or stuffed into sacks in the morning, unrolling them is impossible the next night. The weight that these bags acquire is a direct reflection on the insensible moisture loss of the body during the period of time that they are used. The only exception would be additional water loss from respiration if one were to breath snuggled inside the bags - a technique that we try to avoid.

Sir Charles Wright, a member of the second Scott expedition to the South Pole in 1910 related the problem they had with sleeping bags icing terribly during the trip:

> "When it was cold the bags just filled with ice and that was that. It took an hour to get in. Put your feet in. Melt that much. Shove further."

Sleeping bags gained 30 pounds of ice. They could not be rolled in the morning for they would be impossible to unroll that night. They were loaded onto the sledges flat with clothing stuffed into the opening to provide a starting wedge for getting back into them at night.[1]

In the use of vapor barrier liners for our sleeping bags we have found very little moisture formation inside these liners. In fact, we note a slight sticky feeling to our skin when sleeping naked, with no measurable moisture in the waterproof lining. Wearing polypro underwear made sleeping in the vapor barrier pleasant, once the initial warm-up period of about 2 minutes was passed. Climbing into a plastic bag at colder than -20°F (-28.9°C) is a thrill that anyone could do without, but it certainly proved well worth this effort, for crawling into a solidly frozen bag is much more difficult.

The use of vapor barrier has also been advised for use during bitter cold weather as an undergarment for day use. This requires the wearing of a tight fitting waterproof jacket and pants. The major benefit without doubt is protection of outer clothing from body moisture. Another claimed benefit is decreased dehydration. The severe problem is ventilation of heat. Most work done under bitter winter conditions requires the volitional expenditure of energy with sometimes a considerable amount of heat being generated as indicated elsewhere in this book. While this vapor barrier will prevent sweat from wetting clothing, it is important to not overheat. Sweat must evaporate to help dissipate heat, and the vapor barrier will prevent this. However, simply opening parkas and increasing exposure to bitter cold air will also allow this heat dissipation. Undergarment vapor barrier is not usable except under bitter cold conditions.

I have doubts that there is a decrease in dehydration from the daytime use of vapor barrier under work clothes. Under bitter cold conditions the loss of water through respiration is greatly increased, far beyond the normal percentage of its usual contribution to insensible moisture loss. Especially with heavy exercise, the moisture loss through respiration will negate the slight saving through vapor barrier.

The use of a vapor barrier liner in boot socks works extremely well. It preserves outer socks from foot moisture thus preserving

[1] Source: *"Snow"* by Ruth Kirk, William Morrow & Company, New York 1977

their insulation ability. It is particularly important in protecting felt boot liners. I find it ideal to wear a pair of polypro socks under a vapor barrier sock. Over that one or two pairs of heavy wool socks. Boots should be large enough to accommodate these layers without cramping feet. Constriction of blood flow must be avoided under bitter cold conditions to help prevent frost bite.

The major manufacturers of vapor barrier liners currently are: Patagonia Softwear (Box 150, Ventura, CA 93001); Camp 7 (802 S. Sherman, Longmont, CO 80501); Stephensons Warmlite Equipment, RFD 4, Box 145, Briarcliff Avenue, Gilford, New Hampshire 03246; and Indiana Camp Supply (Box 344F, Pittsboro, IN 46167).

DRESSING FOR COMFORT VS HEAT CONSERVATION

Dr. William Kaufman at the University of Wisconsin in Green Bay has performed significant studies demonstrating that dressing for comfort may not provide proper protection from hypothermic environmental conditions. His work indicates that skin kept too warm would fail to allow various reflex actions to take place, thus lulling the body into a false sense of environmental comfort and allowing a core temperature drop to occur. His experiments do not indicate a profound drop, but the drop of 3.6°F (2°C) indicates a lack of proper energy conservation.

Figure 31 illustrates results from the above experiments. Individuals were dressed in a clothing ensemble that was rated for -26°F (-32°C) exposure. When exposed to that temperature, the core temperature remained fairly steady and generally rose about .9°F (.5°C). When exposed to a lower temperature than the clothing was designed to handle, the core temperature initially rose as vasoconstriction and then shivering attempted to maintain the core temperature level. But the heat loss caused the core temperature to start falling, which it continued to do throughout the time of the experiment. Surprisingly though, upon exposure to a warmer temperature of -14.8°F (-26°C), the core temperature actually fell during the first 150 minutes prior to returning to base line levels. This illustrated the

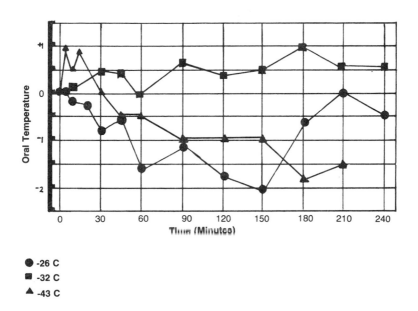

● -26 C
■ -32 C
▲ -43 C

FIGURE 31   "CORE TEMPERATURE DROP FROM IMPROPER INSULATION"
Changes in body sub-lingual temperature when dressed in clothing rated for -25.6°F (-32°C) and
exposed to higher, equivalent, and lower environmental temperatures. Note that when exposed to a
higher temperature (-14.8°F or -26°C), the core readings dropped during the first 150 minutes before
returning to base line at 210 minutes. This is probably due to the warm clothing fooling the
thermoregulation mechanism, thus allowing unnecessary core heat loss. (Adapted from W.C. Kaufman "Cold Weather Clothing for Comfort or Heat Conservation," *Physician and Sportsmedicine*,
February 1982)

lack of thermoregulation on the part of the body when the skin was
too warmly dressed, thus resulting in the core temperature depression. Once the body caught on to the heat loss, central temperature
receptors caused the core temperature depression to be corrected.

Most outdoors travelers have noted that feeling a little coolness
on the extremities is not an unpleasant sensation. This is a reason
that insulated vests make such comfortable additions to the outdoor
clothing wardrobe. By keeping the torso warm and allowing the
arms to cool, the body senses cold weather stress and adequately

compensates to keep core temperatures from falling. This loss of energy stores might be insignificant for a short term exposure and for a long term exposure the eventual correction of body thermal reflexes will apparently prevent a continuous loss. These results might be the most significant for repeated short term exposures to the cold, say leaving and entering a warm work area or cabin, which might fool the body into repeatedly failing to provide adequate thermal protection. It has also been shown experimentally that repeated exposures to cold water and then rapid rewarming would cause a more pronounced drop in core temperature during the cold exposures than would otherwise be experienced. Persons who are going to repetitiously expose themselves for short times to a cold environment should dress so that their trunk is warm, but allow arms, hands, legs and feet to feel somewhat cold.

METALLIZED PLASTIC SHEETS
Their Role and Limitations for Survival and Rescue

The cryogenics industries and the space research activities of NASA resulted in the development of aluminized plastic sheets, or space blankets. These have proven invaluable in the vacuum of space where radiation is the most important aspect of heat exchange. The use of metallized materials has been explored for possible use in the construction of warmer sleeping bags, gloves, and in the production of single and double layer sheets of coated plastic for use in survival situations.

The use of sheets of any material has profound disadvantages in wind. Wind tunnel experiments demonstrate that winds above 20 mph (32 k/hr) make sheeted materials unmanageable. Wrapping a victim in that wind speed can be accomplished only with extreme difficulty. The flapping soon produces gaps in the protection which rapidly carries away the entire sheet. Bags taped together from light weight metallic plastic sheeting were more manageable, but at wind speeds above 20 mph they quickly disintegrated. Bags constructed from polyethylene of .12 mm thickness or greater and ripstop nylon could withstand winds of 40 mph (64 k/hr) even when intentionally punctured.

A Royal Air Force (UK) study of infrared reflection and heat conservation of metallized plastic sheeting *failed to demonstrate any significant difference between using the reflective materials or plain plastic sheeting or ripstop nylon material in their experiments*! Half of their studies were performed at -13°F (-25°C) in still air and half at 17°F (-8°C) in a wind speed of 10 mph (16 k/hr). Skin temperatures were measured with the 8 subjects for each experiment wearing winter clothing and laying at rest. Particularly at the lower temperature, hoar frost rapidly accumulated on the inside of the plastic sheeting which effectively blocked the radiant reflective characteristics of the metallized surface.

The above study would also demonstrate the reduction of a reflective material's ability to return radiant energy to the wearer when that material was woven into or layered within other material. The radiant reflection would be minimized to the point that actual skin difference could be negligible.

A simple experiment demonstrates how the slightest covering of a radiant barrier decreases its ability to prevent radiant heat loss. Two naked humans in close contact will feel a radiant heat from each other. If one wears so much as a thin cotton T-shirt, this radiant heat is remarkably decreased. Conductive heat transfer continues through the T-shirt, which itself will release radiant infrared energy. But a considerable portion of the radiant energy has been absorbed by the T-shirt from the wearer.

A reflective heat barrier may provide minor help when incorporated into clothing and sleeping gear. However, sleeping gear and parkas that incorporate a reflective barrier as part of their design are not increasing the insulating ability significantly with this material. These garments must rely on other design features and the type of insulation fill to provide their significant net insulation effect.

A metallized or plain plastic sheet also serves to protect from convection losses, up to the speed of its vulnerability to flap or wind destruction. It also protects from latent heat of evaporation losses. But it will provide no protection from conduction loss, which in a hypothermia victim can be a very important source of heat loss due to their increased surface area in contact with the ground or other cold surface.

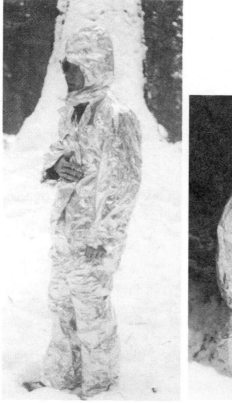
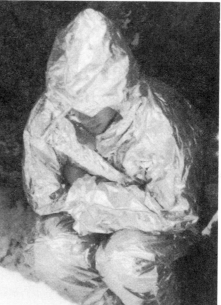

FIGURE 32   "THE COLD WEATHER
SURVIVAL SUIT"
Survival suits of metallized plastic sheeting will
withstand wind conditions above 40 mph (64
k/hr), while it has been shown that tightly tucked
sheets will flap apart at winds of 20 mph (32
k/hr). These suits are available through many
outdoor outfitters.

7. OTHER COLD RELATED INJURIES
Frostbite

Frostbite is the freezing of tissue. Surface skin goes through several phases before this occurs. The freezing process requires predisposing risk factors to be present before the events leading to frostbite are initiated.

Outside temperatures must be below freezing for frostbite to occur. The underlying physical condition of the victim, length of cold contact, and type of cold contact are other important factors leading to frostbite. Skin temperature must be cooled to between 22°F to 24°F (-5.5°C to -4.4°C) before tissue will freeze.

A decreased peripheral circulation from vasoconstriction due to hypothermia can be an important factor in frostbite formation, but generally even severe vasoconstriction will not be enough unless one of several other situations are present.

One is the wearing of constricting garments, such as boots that are too tight, or elastic wrist or ankle bands that are too snug. Boot liners constructed of foam material with air cells that can expand at high altitude have caused many frostbitten feet in mountaineers. Cold weather clothing should be constructed to avoid constricting bands on ankles and wrists especially.

Dehydration is a risk factor for frostbite. As indicated elsewhere, dehydration is also a risk factor for hypothermia. Dehydration will generally exist in a person suffering from chronic hypothermia.

Adequate nutrition and prevention of fatigue are additional preventative measures in the fight against frostbite. This is in large measure due to their importance in preventing hypothermia.

It is rare for a healthy person, even with reduced activity in bitter cold weather - such as encountered with prolonged standing - to develop frostbite. But injury of any sort seems to allow frostbite to more easily develop. If shock is present, the risk of frostbite injury increases dramatically.

Contact with metal objects which rapidly conduct heat from the body may cause frostbite. Even a thin glove which, while allowing dexterity and not providing much insulation, would be valuable in preventing direct contact with metal hardware used in climbing, work, or camping under below freezing situations. Extreme caution with liquid fuels must be maintained as these liquids will cool to the recent average ambient temperature and will cause immediate tissue freezing in subzero conditions.

The use of substances that cause vasoconstriction, primarily smoking, should be avoided. In healthy people smoking does not appear to cause increased risk of frostbite as long as they are not smoking during the time of cold exposure. Persons sensitive to the effects of nicotine, such as those suffering from Raynaud's or Buerger's disease, must absolutely quit smoking and are at risk of frostbite during freezing conditions.

Lack of adequate oxygen supply is also a factor. This is much more prevalent in high altitude climbing. It is particularly noticeable that climbing above 24,500 feet (7,500 meters) without oxygen frequently results in extensive frostbite amongst even highly experienced climbling parties.

Of all of the factors mentioned, hypothermia itself is the most imporant predisposing factor to the formation of frostbite. But a person with hypothermia may well not have frostbite, and vice-versa, a person with frostbite may not be hypothermic.

Generally when frostbite occurs, it will be to feet, hands, ears, or nose. Only rarely will it occur elsewhere and then only with some unusual cause, such as metal contact, injury, etc.

As mentioned elsewhere, an important method of body heat control is the vasoconstriction of arteries to prevent warm blood flow to the surface and thus decrease heat loss. In the skin, the heat and oxygen transfer occurs in the capillary system, the microscopic vessels that connect the veins and arteries together. These thin vessels are so small, that red blood cells must travel through them in single file. When the small peripheral arteries, called arterioles, clamp down, the blood flow to the capillaries ceases. Blood is shunted from the arterioles directly to small veins, venules. Oxygen and heat is no longer provided local tissue, carbon dioxide and waste products are no longer removed. The "hunting reflex" (see page 51) can allow periodic surges of warm blood through the arteriole-venule shunt to provide a certain amount of local heat to help prevent tissue freezing. But if the body core temperature drops, this episodic warming will decrease to the point that local tissue freezing may result.

If the outside temperature is below freezing, and the circulation of warm blood has been compromised, the fluid between the cells may start to freeze. This freezing process pulls additional fluid from the surrounding cells as the ice crystals grow. While these crystals do not seem to cause tissue damage, the dehydration process results in damage to the cell's internal metabolic systems and structures. This damage can become severe within half an hour. In the case of rapid freezing, say from contact with metal or liquid fuels during bitter cold temperatures, ice crystal formation can occur both between cells and within the cells, thus more rapidly destroying these cells and preventing any chance of recovery of this injured tissue.

Traditionally several degrees of frostbite are recognized, but the initial treatment for all is the same. The actual degree of severity will not be known for an extended period of time.

By definition frostbite means that tissue has been not only frozen, but damaged (see frost nip on page 110). For practical purposes, two types of frostbite are generally recognized, although some authorities go as far as 4 degrees. The first type is "superficial frostbite". The surface layer of skin is frozen, but deeper tissues are not. When pressing on a superficial frostbite it will be noted that while the surface is frozen and white, it will give under firm, gentle pressure as lower tissues are still pliable. In the second type, "deep frostbite," even the deeper tissues are frozen solid. This tissue feels hard as a rock. There will be considerable chance for full recovery of tissue with superficial frostbite, while deep frostbite can result in considerable tissue destruction.

Once thawing has taken place, it will be impossible to use the above criteria for distinguishing superficial from deep frostbite. After thawing, the formation of blisters may be a guide as to the severity of the freeze damage and can act as a prognosis as to the eventual damage that may result. If the blisters form within 24 to 36 hours and are located towards the tips of the fingers or toes, the damage was most likely superficial. Blisters that take 3 to 7 days to form and those located further up the hand or leg generally indicate severe peripheral damage and the tissue beyond that point may be dead with eventual total loss.

The specific therapy for a deep frozen extremity is rapid thawing in warm water of approximately 110°F (43.3°C). Take precautions to never let this water temperature be higher than 115°F (46°C) or the results will be disastrous. This thawing may take 20 to 30 minutes. It should be continued until all paleness of the tips of the toes or fingers has turned to pink or burgundy red, but no longer. This will be very painful and will require pain medication at the start of the procedure. Frostbite victims should be treated for shock routinely with elevation of the feet and lowering of the head, as shock can easily occur when the frostbite victim enters a warm environment.

Avoid opening the blisters that form. Do not cut the skin away, but allow the blisters to eventually resolve on their own. These blisters will usually last 2 to 3 weeks. They must be treated with care to prevent infections (best done in a hospital with gloved attendants). The worse complication that can develop at this stage is an infection of these tissues, resulting in a "wet gangrene." Infection can cause considerable tissue loss, far beyond the area of initial freeze injury. It is important that the patient's tetanus immunization be current, certainly within the previous 10 years.

A black carapace will form in severe frostbite. This is actually a form of dry gangrene. This carapace will gradually fall off with amazingly good results beneath. Efforts to hasten carapace removal generally result in infection, delay in healing, and increased loss of tissue. Leave these blackened areas alone. The black carapace separation can take over 6 months, but it is worth the wait. Without surgical intervention most frostbite wounds heal in six months to a year. At times emergency surgery *is* indicated in freeze injuries. After thawing, tissue swelling can become so profound that the remaining circulation may be compromised. Surgery to relieve this pressure, called a ''fasciotomy,'' must be performed. The necessity for this procedure is indicated by sophisticated methods of blood flow and tissue pressure analysis.

If a frozen member has been thawed and the patient must be transported, use cotton between toes (or fluff sterile gauze and place between the toes) and cover other areas with a loose sterile bandage to protect the skin during sleeping bag/stretcher evacuation. If a fracture also exists, immobilize when in the field, loosely so as not to impair the circulation any further.

It is important to note that refreezing will result in substantial tissue loss. The frozen part should not be thawed if there is any possibility of refreezing the part. Also, once the victim has undergone thawing, very careful management of the thawed part and the patient is required. The patient actually becomes a stretcher case if the foot is involved. For that reason it may be necessary to leave the foot or leg(s) frozen and allow the victim to walk back to the evacuation point or facility where the thawing will take place.

Peter Freuchen, the great Greenland explorer, once walked days and miles keeping one leg frozen, knowing that when his leg thawed he would be helpless. The longer tissue is kept frozen, the less likely it can be thawed without damage, but refreezing thawed tissue is certain disaster and must be avoided. The decision to continue hiking on a frostbitten foot is a serious one, as additional tissue loss may result. Lying in the field awaiting evacuation that would unduly prolong treatment, or perhaps expose the victim and other party members to hypothermia or further frostbite injury, is an equally serious decision. The correct approach to this situation will depend upon numerous local circumstances, but at least be aware of the potential results of each decision. Peter Freuchen's full length portrait in the Explorers Club building in New York City, showing his peg leg, is a potent reminder of the dangers of frostbite for even a highly experienced arctic explorer.

Frost Nip

Frost nip, or superficial surface freezing, can be readily treated in the field, if recognized early enough. By watching for, and immediately responding to frost nip, permanent damage to tissue can be avoided.

Frost nip is most common on the ears and the tip of the nose. When frost nip is suspected, thaw immediately so that it does not become a more serious frostbite. Warm the hands by blowing on them, placing them as fists within mittens, or withdrawing them into the parka through the sleeves -- avoid opening the front of the parka to minimize heat loss.

It is difficult to evaluate the existence of frost nip on feet. A good clue is the loss of sensation in the toes and foot, which should mandate examination if sensation cannot be readily restored by increasing activity or stomping of the feet. Feet should be thawed against a companion or cupped in your own hands in a roomy sleeping bag, or otherwise placed in contact with warm human flesh in an insulated environment.

Your own nose can be thawed by cupping your hands over your face and exhaling. Ears can be warmed by pressing warm hands over them. Your hands may have to be warmed first by blowing on them or insulating them adequately in large mittens, etc.

Frost nip can be painless and its presence should be watched for on your companions. It is seldom encountered; however on one of my winter trips into sub-arctic Canada, a companion almost constantly frost nipped his nose whenever the temperature fell below -20°F (-29°C). He was healthy, in excellent physical shape (probably the best conditioned of us all), and he wore arctic clothing that was identical to the rest of ours. We repeatedly had to warn him to thaw his nose, as he seemed oblivious to the fact that the tip of his nose was literally frosted white.

Frozen Lung

A condition called frozen lung, or more properly "pulmonary chilling," as no tissue is actually frozen, may occur when breathing rapidly at very low temperatures, generally colder than -20°F (-29°C). There is burning pain, sometimes coughing of blood, and frequently asthmatic wheezing. If irritation of the diaphragm occurs, a pain in the shoulder(s) and upper stomach may develop which can last for 1 to 2 weeks.

The cause of this condition is a severe bronchial irritation. This results in bronchospams, the formation of mucous, and possibly pulmonary infiltration resulting in the pleuritic pain.

The treatment is bed rest, steam inhalations, drinking extra water, humidification of the air being breathed, and absolutely no smoking. This problem may be avoided by using parka hoods, face masks or breathing through mufflers which allow the rebreathing of warm humidified, expired air.

Immersion Foot

Immersion foot, also called "trench foot," results during wet, cold conditions with temperature exposures from 68°F (20°C) down to freezing, if proper foot care is not maintained. It results from vasoconstriction of the arterioles with subsequent loss of heat and oxygen supply to surface tissues. Under prolonged exposure to wet, cold conditions, this can result in damage to the skin. The temperature need not drop below 50°F (10°C) for substantial injury to occur.

To prevent this problem avoid non-breathing (rubber) footwear when possible. Dry feet and change socks when feet get wet or sweaty every 3 to 4 hours, if necessary. Periodically elevate, air, dry, massage the feet to promote circulation. Avoid tight, constricting footwear or lower leg garments.

One might question the possible development of immersion foot when using a vapor barrier sock (page 99). I do not know if this has ever occurred, but it is a possibility. My companions and I have never found our liner socks to be very damp, but a mountaineering friend of mine reports wringing considerable water from his liner socks when using a vapor barrier system. In that instance, the main protection from immersion foot injury would be the maintenance of a very warm foot, made possible from the superior or protected insulation. The U.S. Army "mickey mouse" or "bunny" boots used under arctic conditions allow considerable moisture build-up. These boots are generally very warm, thus precluding the formation of immersion foot. But a precaution everyone should take when using an occlusive boot or liner system, is to dry feet nightly and sooner if they feel cold.

There are two stages of immersion foot clinically. In the first stage the foot is cold, swollen, waxy, mottled with dark burgundy to blue splotches. This foot is resilient to palpation, whereas the frozen foot is very hard. Skin is sodden and friable. Loss of feeling makes walking difficult.

The second stage lasts for days to weeks. The feet become swollen, red and hot. Blisters form, infection and gangrene are frequently problems during this stage.

Treatment differs from frostbite and hypothermia in the following ways: 1) Give the patient 10 grains of aspirin every 6 hours to help decrease platelet adhesion and clotting ability of the blood; 2) Give additional stronger pain medication if necessary, but discontinue as soon as possible; 3) Provide an ounce of hard liquor (30 ml) every hour while awake and 2 ounces (60 ml) every 2 hours during sleeping hours to vasodilate and increase the blood flow to the feet.

If you are unsure whether or not you are dealing with immersion foot or frostbite, or if you may have suffered both, treat as for frostbite. The injury of immersion foot should be treated by a physician. The chance of damaging the tissue, or serious infection, and of long term pain and other complications is very high.

Chilblain

Chilblain, also commonly called "pernio," and less frequently "kibe" and "chimetlon," results from exposure of dry skin to temperatures from 60°F (15.5°C) to freezing. The skin becomes red, swollen, frequently tender and itching. This is the least severe form of cold injury. No tissue loss ever results. Strictly speaking, the term "kibe" refers to a crack in the skin caused by cold or an ulcerated chilblain.

The cause is probably histamine release in cold traumatized tissue, resulting in further tissue irritation.

Treatment is the prevention of further exposure with protective clothing over bare skin and the use of ointments such as A & D Ointment or Vaseline (white petrolatum).

Appendix I

STATE OF ALASKA
Guidelines for the Management of
HYPOTHERMIA
and
COLD WATER NEAR DROWNING

The Guidelines listed in this appendix have been adapted for use by medical personnel in Alaska and have been published by State of Alaska, Department of Health and Social Services, Division of Public Health, Emergency Medical Services Section, and are presented here with their kind permission.

These guidelines are the result of a conference on hypothermia and cold water near drowning held in Anchorage, Alaska, on 11 and 12 July 1981. Moderating the conference was Tim Samuelson, M.D. Also participating were William Doolittle, M.D., John Hayward, Ph.D., William Mills, M.D., and Martin Nemiroff, M.D.

They have been developed for use by prehospital and hospital personnel dealing with cold problems in Alaska. They are meant to be guidelines, not absolute rules, governing the treatment of hypothermia and cold water near drowning.

They do not address the treatment of frostbite, which has been covered in the text on pages 108-110. For further management techniques of hypothermia and immersion injuries, see pages 51-77. Immersion foot treatment is on page 112.

HYPOTHERMIA:
GENERAL POINTS

A. The evaluation and treatment of hypothermia whether wet or dry, on land or water, is essentially the same. Therefore, the following discussion does not specifically distinguish between chronic and acute, or wet and dry hypothermia.

B. In the cold patient, a rectal temperature is one of the vital signs. In terms of the ABC's, think:

    A — Airway
    B — Breathing
    C — Circulation
    D — Degrees

C. "Low Reading" thermometers are important in the care of the hypothermic patient. Regular thermometers are useless and probably dangerous in this setting.

D. Obtaining a temperature is important and useful for treating hypothermia. However, there is tremendous variability in individual physiologic responses at specific temperatures. In addition, there will be times when a low reading thermometer is not available. Therefore, these guidelines are not based on the patient's measured temperature.

E. Axiom: With the hypothermic patient, THINK HEAT.
    1. No cold I.V.'s
    2. No cold ventilation therapy.
    3. No cold treatments of any kind.

F. Unheated oxygen should not be used for the hypothermia victim because it will add cold to the victim. Attempt to administer warm, moist oxygen if possible.

G. We must, at least, <u>prevent further heat loss at the core</u>. This can only be done by insulating the entire patient, plus adding heat to the "core areas" (head, neck, chest and groin).

H. <u>Add heat</u> gradually and gently:

(The term "add heat" is used rather than "rewarm" because often the patient is not actually any warmer with the addition of heat, but rather only a further decrease in core temperature is minimized.)

   1. Apply external warm objects to the head, neck, chest and groin. Use:

      a. Hot water bottles.

      b. "Warm packs" (chemical heat packs must be used with great care so as not to burn the patient's skin, e.g. wrap in a towel and watch carefully).

      c. Warm rocks wrapped in towels.

      d. Warm bodies, etc.

   2. Administer warm, moist air or oxygen.

I. Do not ever try to cool the extremities or use tourniquets or other occlusive dressings.

J. Be wary of statements or actions while working on patients who are unconscious or requiring CPR. These patients frequently remember what is done and said and it can produce severe psychological problems later on. This statement applies equally well to warm and cold patients.

K. It is absolutely necessary that you pre-plan how you will handle these problems and who will be in charge; and that you are familiar with the appropriate equipment.

L. A note on transport: Air travel in Alaska is obviously favored. But, if air travel is not possible, other types of transport should be utilized, such as snowmachines, dog teams, cars, and especially boats in areas with water access.

M. The inside of the ambulance and any rooms where such patients are treated should be "room temperature" — approximately 65 to 72 degrees F. [18 to 22 degrees C.].

HYPOTHERMIA:
FIRST RESPONDER / GENERAL PUBLIC

A. Assessment of Patient

1. Severe Hypothermia: If the victim is cold and has any of the following signs or symptoms, he is considered to have severe hypothermia:

a. Depressed vital signs.

b. Altered level of consciousness, including slurred speech, staggering gait, decreased mental skills.

c. Temperature of 90 degrees F. (32 degrees C.) or less.

d. No shivering in spite of being very cold. (Note: This sign may be altered by alcohol intoxication.)

e. Associated significant illness or injury that is present or that may have permitted the hypothermia to develop.

2. Mild to Moderate Hypothermia: If the victim is cold and does not have any of these signs or symptoms, he is considered to have mild to moderate hypothermia.

B.   Basic Treatment for Hypothermia

1.   Treat very gently.

2.   Remove wet clothing. Replace with dry clothing or dry coverings of some kind.

3.   Insulate from the cold.

4.   Add heat to the head, neck, chest and groin externally (see H under "General Points" on page 117), or internally, if a system for breathing warm moist air is available. Avoid attempts to warm the extremities.

     Note: In reality, when prehospital personnel add heat, they rarely actually raise the core temperature. Rather, they succeed in preventing a further decrease in core temperature. If the core temperature in a very cold patient were raised significantly, electrolyte, acid-base and dehydration problems could occur.

5.   Do not rub or manipulate the extremities.

6.   Do not give coffee or alcohol.

7.   Do not put patient in a shower or bath.

8.   Warm fluids can be given only after uncontrollable shivering stops and the victim has a clear level of consciousness, the ability to swallow, and evidence of rewarming already.

9.   If severe hypothermia is present, treat as above and transport to a higher medical facility.

10. If there is no way to get to a higher medical facility, rewarm the patient slowly, cautiously and gradually with methods indicated in H under "General Points" on page 117.

C. Treatment for Severe Hypothermia with No Life Signs
   (CPR Required)

   1. Provide basic treatment as indicated in Section B above.

   2. Carefully assess the presence or absence of pulse or respirations for one to two minutes.

   3. If no pulse or respirations, start CPR.

   4. Use mouth-to-mouth rather than bag/mask breathing.

   5. Obtain a rectal temperature if possible.

   6. If you are less than 15 minutes to a higher medical facility, do not bother trying to add heat.

   7. If you are greater than 15 minutes to a higher medical facility, add heat gradually and gently (see Section H under "General Points" on page 117).

   8. Reassess the physical status periodically.

   9. Transfer to a higher medical facility in all cases.

HYPOTHERMIA: FIRST RESPONDER/GENERAL PUBLIC

D. Treatment for Severe Hypothermia with Signs of Life (i.e.
    Pulse and Respirations Present; CPR Not Required)

    1. Provide treatment as indicated in Section B above.

    2. If you are greater than 15 minutes to a higher medical
        facility, add heat gradually and gently (see Section H
        under "General Points" on page 117).

    3. Transfer to a higher medical facility.

HYPOTHERMIA:
EMERGENCY MEDICAL TECHNICIAN I*

A. Assessment of Patient

    1. Severe Hypothermia: If the victim is cold and has <u>any</u> of
        the following signs or symptoms, he is considered to have
        severe hypothermia:

        a. Depressed vital signs.

        b. Altered level of consciousness, including slurred
            speech, staggering gait, decreased mental skills.

        c. Temperature of 90 degrees F. (32 degrees C.) or less.

        d. No shivering in spite of being very cold. (Note: This
            sign may be altered by alcohol intoxication.)

        e. Associated significant illness or injury that is present
            or that may have permitted the hypothermia to de-
            velop.

    2. Mild to Moderate Hypothermia: If the victim is cold and
        does not have any of these signs or symptoms, he is
        considered to have mild to moderate hypothermia.

        *In Alaska, Community Health Aides, for the purposes
        of these protocols, are considered to fall into this category.

B.   Basic Treatment for Hypothermia

1.   Treat very gently.

2.   Remove wet clothing. Replace with dry clothing or dry coverings of some kind.

3.   Insulate from the cold.

4.   Add heat to the head, neck, chest and groin externally (see H under "General Points" on page 117), or internally, if a system for breathing warm moist air is available. Avoid attempts to warm the extremities.

     Note: In reality, when prehospital personnel add heat, they rarely actually raise the core temperature. Rather, they succeed in preventing a further decrease in core temperature. If the core temperature in a very cold patient were raised significantly, electrolyte, acid-base and dehydration problems could occur.

5.   Do not rub or manipulate the extremities.

6.   Do not give coffee or alcohol.

7.   Do not put patient in a shower or bath.

8.   Warm fluids can be given only after uncontrollable shivering stops and the victim has a clear level of consciousness, the ability to swallow, and evidence of rewarming already.

9.   Communicate with a higher medical facility.

10.   If severe hypothermia is present, treat as above and transport to a higher medical facility.

11.   If there is no way to get to a higher medical facility, rewarm the patient slowly, cautiously and gradually with methods indicated in H under "General Points" on page 117.

C.

Additional Therapy

1. Do not use oxygen unless you are performing CPR or you are specifically told to do so.

2. The indications for oral airways are the same in both the hypothermic and the warm patient.

3. Pneumatic antishock garments are not indicated for hypothermia, but may be used to treat hypovolemic shock in a hypothermic patient.

D Treatment for Severe Hypothermia with No Life Signs CPR Required)

1. Provide basic and additional treatment as indicated in Sections B and C above.

2. Carefully assess the presence or absence of pulse or respirations for one to two minutes.

3. If no pulse or respirations, start CPR.

4. Use mouth-to-mouth rather than bag/mask breathing.

5. Use oxygen, oral airways, or pneumatic antishock garments as indicated in Section C above.

6. Obtain a rectal temperature if possible.

7. Communicate with a higher medical facility.

8. If you are less than 15 minutes to a higher medical facility, do not bother trying to add heat.

9.   If you are greater than 15 minutes to a higher medical facility, add heat gradually and gently (see Section H under ''General Points'' on page 117).

10.   Reassess the physical status periodically.

11.   Transfer to a higher medical facility <u>in all cases</u>.

E.   <u>Treatment for Severe Hypothermia with Signs of Life (i.e. Pulse and Respirations Present; CPR Not Required)</u>

1.   Provide basic and additional treatment as indicated in Sections B and C above.

2.   If you are greater than 15 minutes to a higher medical facility, add heat gradually and gently (see Section H under ''General Points'' on page 117).

3.   Transfer to a higher medical facility.

HYPOTHERMIA:
EMERGENCY MEDICAL TECHNICIAN II

A. Assessment of Patient

    1.   Severe Hypothermia: If the victim is cold and has <u>any</u> of the following signs or symptoms, he is considered to have severe hypothermia:

        a.   Depressed vital signs.

        b.   Altered level of consciousness, including slurred speech, staggering gait, decreased mental skills.

        c.   Temperature of 90 degrees F. (32 degrees C.) or less.

        d.   No shivering in spite of being very cold. (Note: This sign may be altered by alcohol intoxication.)

        e.   Associated significant illness or injury that is present or that may have permitted the hypothermia to develop.

    2.   Mild to Moderate Hypothermia: If the victim is cold and does not have any of these signs or symptoms, he is considered to have mild to moderate hypothermia.

B. Basic Treatment for Hypothermia

   1. Treat very gently.

   2. Remove wet clothing. Replace with dry clothing or dry coverings of some kind.

   3. Insulate from the cold.

   4. Add heat to the head, neck, chest and groin externally (see H under "General Points" on page 117), or internally, if a system for breathing warm moist air is available. Avoid attempts to warm the extremities.

      Note: In reality, when prehospital personnel add heat, they rarely actually raise the core temperature. Rather, they succeed in preventing a further decrease in core temperature. If the core temperature in a very cold patient were raised significantly, electrolyte, acid-base and dehydration problems could occur.

   5. Do not rub or manipulate the extremities.

   6. Do not give coffee or alcohol.

   7. Do not put patient in a shower or bath.

   8. Warm fluids can be given only after uncontrollable shivering stops and the victim has a clear level of consciousness, the ability to swallow, and evidence of rewarming already.

   9. Communicate with a higher medical facility.

   10. If severe hypothermia is present, treat as above and transport to a higher medical facility.

   11. If there is no way to get to a higher medical facility, rewarm the patient slowly, cautiously and gradually with methods indicated in H under "General Points" on page 117.

C.

Additional Therapy

1. Do not use oxygen unless you are performing CPR or you are specifically told to do so.

2. The indications for oral airways are the same in both the hypothermic and the warm patient.

3. The Esophageal Airway Device: The indications and contraindications for the esophageal airway device are the same in both the hypothermic and the warm patient.

4. Pneumatic antishock garments are not indicated for hypothermia, but may be used to treat hypovolemic shock in a hypothermic patient.

5. I.V. Therapy:
    a. Do not delay transport, communications, or other therapy by taking a long time to start an I.V. I.V.'s are difficult to start in cold patients.
    b. All patients with severe hypothermia should have an I.V. started after other stabilization.
    c. Use D_5W at a rate of 75 cc's per hour.

6. Medications:
    a. Medications are inefficient and poorly metabolized in the hypothermic patient.
    b. Narcan, 50% Dextrose, and Sodium Bicarbonate are not to be used unless specifically ordered by a physician.

D. Treatment for Severe Hypothermia with No Life Signs
    CPR Required)

    1. Provide basic and additional treatment as indicated in
        Sections B and C above.

    2. Carefully assess the presence or absence of pulse or respi-
        rations for one to two minutes.

    3. If no pulse or respirations, start CPR.

    4. Use mouth-to-mouth rather than bag/mask breathing.

    5. Use oxygen, oral airways, esophageal airway devices,
        pneumatic antishock garments, I.V.'s, and medications
        as indicated in Section C above.

    6. Obtain a rectal temperature if possible.

    7. Communicate with a higher medical facility.

    8. If you are less than 15 minutes to a higher medical facility,
        do not bother trying to add heat.

    9. If you are greater than 15 minutes to a higher medical
        facility, add heat gradually and gently (see Section H
        under "General Points" on page 117).

    10. Reassess the physical status periodically.

    11. Transfer to a higher medical facility in all cases.

E. Treatment for Severe Hypothermia with Signs of Life (i.e. Pulse and Respirations Present; CPR Not Required)

1. Provide basic and additional treatment as indicated in Sections B and C above.

2. If you are greater than 15 minutes to a higher medical facility, add heat gradually and gently (see Section H under "General Points" on page 117).

3. Transfer to a higher medical facility.

HYPOTHERMIA:
EMERGENCY MEDICAL TECHNICIAN III

A. Assessment of Patient

    1. <u>Severe Hypothermia</u>: If the victim is cold and has <u>any</u> of the following signs or symptoms, he is considered to have severe hypothermia:

        a. Depressed vital signs.

        b. Altered level of consciousness, including slurred speech, staggering gait, decreased mental skills.

        c. Temperature of 90 degrees F. (32 degrees C.) or less.

        d. No shivering in spite of being very cold. (Note: This sign may be altered by alcohol intoxication.)

        e. Associated significant illness or injury that is present or that may have permitted the hypothermia to develop.

    2. <u>Mild to Moderate Hypothermia</u>: If the victim is cold and does not have any of these signs or symptoms, he is considered to have mild to moderate hypothermia.

B. Basic Treatment for Hypothermia

    1.   Treat very gently.

    2.   Remove wet clothing. Replace with dry clothing or dry coverings of some kind.

    3.   Insulate from the cold.

    4.   Add heat to the head, neck, chest and groin externally (see H under "General Points" on page 117), or internally, if a system for breathing warm moist air is available. Avoid attempts to warm the extremities.

        Note: In reality, when prehospital personnel add heat, they rarely actually raise the core temperature. Rather, they succeed in preventing a further decrease in core temperature. If the core temperature in a very cold patient were raised significantly, electrolyte, acid-base and dehydration problems could occur.

    5.   Do not rub or manipulate the extremities.

    6.   Do not give coffee or alcohol.

    7.   Do not put patient in a shower or bath.

    8.   Warm fluids can be given only after uncontrollable shivering stops and the victim has a clear level of consciousness, the ability to swallow, and evidence of rewarming already.

    9.   Communicate with a higher medical facility.

    10.   If severe hypothermia is present, treat as above and transport to a higher medical facility.

    11.   If there is no way to get to a higher medical facility, rewarm the patient slowly, cautiously and gradually with methods indicated in H under "General Points" on page 117.

C.

Additional Therapy

1. Do not use oxygen unless you are performing CPR or you are specifically told to do so.

2. The indications for oral airways are the same in both the hypothermic and the warm patient.

3. The Esophageal Airway Device: The indications and contraindications for the esophageal airway device are the same in both the hypothermic and the warm patient.

4. Pneumatic antishock garments are not indicated for hypothermia, but may be used to treat hypovolemic shock in a hypothermic patient.

5. I.V. Therapy:
    a. Do not delay transport, communications, or other therapy by taking a long time to start an I.V.   I.V.'s are difficult to start in cold patients.
    b. All patients with severe hypothermia should have an I.V. started after other stabilization.
    c. Use D_5W at a rate of 75 cc's per hour.

6. Medications:
    a. Medications are inefficient and poorly metabolized in the hypothermic patient.
    b. Narcan, 50% Dextrose, and Sodium Bicarbonate are not to be used unless specifically ordered by a physician.
    c. Morphine is contraindicated in the hypothermic patient.
    d. Lidocaine: See Section D.7 below.

7. Cardiac monitoring is indicated in all hypothermic patients as long as its use does not unnecessarily delay other or further care.

D. Treatment for Severe Hypothermia with No Life Signs
    CPR Required)

1. Provide basic and additional treatment as indicated in Sections B and C above.

2. Carefully assess the presence or absence of pulse or respirations for one to two minutes.

3. If no pulse or respirations, start CPR.

4. Use mouth-to-mouth rather than bag/mask breathing.

5. If patient is in ventricular fibrillation or ventricular tachycardia, attempt D/C cardioversion once with 400 w/s's. Note: Shivering can mimic ventricular fibrillation.

6. Repeat cardioversion may be attempted only if the core temperature is 85 degrees F. (30 degrees C.) or higher.

7. If cardioversion is successful, give Lidocaine, approximately 1 mg. per kilogram I.V. bolus, followed in 15 minutes by a second bolus at 0.5 mg per kilogram.

8. If heart rhythm is asystole, do not attempt defibrillation. Treat as an EMT II.

9. Use oxygen, oral airways, esophageal airway devices, pneumatic antishock garments, I.V.'s, and medications and cardiac monitoring as indicated in Section C above.

10. Obtain a rectal temperature if possible.

11. Communicate with a higher medical facility.

12. If you are less than 15 minutes to a higher medical facility, do not bother trying to add heat.

13. If you are greater than 15 minutes to a higher medical facility, add heat gradually and gently (see Section H under "General Points" on page 117).

14. Reassess the physical status periodically.

15. Transfer to a higher medical facility in all cases.

HYPOTHERMIA: EMERGENCY MEDICAL TECHNICIAN III

E.   Treatment for Severe Hypothermia with Signs of Life (i.e.
     Pulse and Respirations Present; CPR Not Required)

     1.   Provide basic and additional treatment as indicated in
          Sections B and C above.

     2.   If you are greater than 15 minutes to a higher medical
          facility, add heat gradually and gently (see Section H
          under "General Points" on page 117).

     3.   Transfer to a higher medical facility.

HYPOTHERMIA: PARAMEDIC

A. Paramedic Role

Paramedics in isolated areas of Alaska should function as EMT IIIs with hypothermic patients, unless they are under the specific on-line direction of a physician, or until a patient reaches a level of adequate physiological response (temperature higher than 90 degrees F).

B. Assessment of Patient

1. Severe Hypothermia: If the victim is cold and has any of the following signs or symptoms, he is considered to have severe hypothermia:

    a. Depressed vital signs.

    b. Altered level of consciousness, including slurred speech, staggering gait, decreased mental skills.

    c. Temperature of 90 degrees F. (32 degrees C.) or less.

    d. No shivering in spite of being very cold. (Note: This sign may be altered by alcohol intoxication.)

    e. Associated significant illness or injury that is present or that may have permitted the hypothermia to develop.

2. Mild to Moderate Hypothermia: If the victim is cold and does not have any of these signs or symptoms, he is considered to have mild to moderate hypothermia.

C. <u>Basic Treatment for Hypothermia</u>

1. Treat very gently.

2. Remove wet clothing. Replace with dry clothing or dry coverings of some kind.

3. Insulate from the cold.

4. Add heat to the head, neck, chest and groin externally (see H under ''General Points'' on page 117), or internally, if a system for breathing warm moist air is available. Avoid attempts to warm the extremities.

    <u>Note</u>: In reality, when prehospital personnel add heat, they rarely actually raise the core temperature. Rather, they succeed in preventing a further decrease in core temperature. If the core temperature in a <u>very</u> cold patient were raised significantly, electrolyte, acid-base and dehydration problems could occur.

5. Do not rub or manipulate the extremities.

6. Do not give coffee or alcohol.

7. Do not put patient in a shower or bath.

8. Warm fluids can be given only after uncontrollable shivering stops and the victim has a clear level of consciousness, the ability to swallow, and evidence of rewarming already.

9. Communicate with a higher medical facility.

10. If <u>severe hypothermia</u> is present, treat as above and transport to a higher medical facility.

11. If there is no way to get to a higher medical facility, rewarm the patient slowly, cautiously and gradually with methods indicated in H under ''General Points'' on page 117.

D.

Additional Therapy

1. Do not use oxygen unless you are performing CPR or you are specifically told to do so.

2. The indications for oral airways are the same in both the hypothermic and the warm patient.

3. The Esophageal Airway Device: The indications and contraindications for the esophageal airway device are the same in both the hypothermic and the warm patient.

4. Endotracheal Intubation: The indications and contraindications for ET tube placement are the same in both the hypothermic and the warm patient.

5. Pneumatic antishock garments are not indicated for hypothermia, but may be used to treat hypovolemic shock in a hypothermic patient.

6. I.V. Therapy:
    a. Do not delay transport, communications, or other therapy by taking a long time to start an I.V.   I.V.'s are difficult to start in cold patients.
    b. All patients with severe hypothermia should have an I.V. started after other stabilization.
    c. Use D_5W at a rate of 75 cc's per hour.

7. Medications:
    a. Since medications are inefficient and poorly metabolized in the hypothermic patient, none of the additional medications utilized by paramedics are indicated, unless specifically ordered by a physician.
    b. Lidocaine: See Section E.7 below.

8. Cardiac monitoring is indicated in all hypothermic patients as long as its use does not unnecessarily delay other or further care.

E. Treatment for Severe Hypothermia with No Life Signs
    CPR Required)

1. Provide basic and additional treatment as indicated in
    Sections B and C above.

2. Carefully assess the presence or absence of pulse or respi-
    rations for one to two minutes.

3. If no pulse or respirations, start CPR.

4. Use mouth-to-mouth rather than bag/mask breathing.

5. If patient is in ventricular fibrillation or ventricular
    tachycardia, attempt D/C cardioversion once with 400
    w/s's. Note: Shivering can mimic ventricular fibrillation.

6. Repeat cardioversion may be attempted only if the core
    temperature is 85 degrees F. (30 degrees C.) or higher.

7. If cardioversion is successful, give Lidocaine, approxi-
    mately 1 mg. per kilogram I.V. bolus, followed in 15
    minutes by a second bolus at 0.5 mg per kilogram.

8. If heart rhythm is asystole, do not attempt defibrillation.
    Treat as an EMT II.

9. Use oxygen, oral airways, esophageal airway devices,
    pneumatic antishock garments, I.V.'s, and medications
    and cardiac monitoring as indicated in Section D above.

10. Obtain a rectal temperature if possible.

11. Communicate with a higher medical facility.

12. If you are less than 15 minutes to a higher medical facility,
    do not bother trying to add heat.

13. If you are greater than 15 minutes to a higher medical
    facility, add heat gradually and gently (see Section H
    under "General Points" on page 117).

14. Reassess the physical status periodically.

15. Transfer to a higher medical facility in all cases.

F. Treatment for Severe Hypothermia with Signs of Life (i.e. Pulse and Respirations Present; CPR Not Required)

1. Provide basic and additional treatment as indicated in Sections C and D above.

2. If you are greater than 15 minutes to a higher medical facility, add heat gradually and gently (see Section H under "General Points" on page 117).

3. Transfer to a higher medical facility.

HYPOTHERMIA: PARAMEDIC

HYPOTHERMIA:
SMALL/BUSH CLINIC

A. The extent of the evaluation and treatment in small/bush clinics
    is defined by the training of the personnel and the available
    equipment as outlined in the foregoing guidelines.

B. For transfer to a higher medical facility, the patient must be
    stabilized in the clinic rather than transferred as an unstable
    patient. If the patient is requiring CPR or is otherwise with
    unstable vital signs, then the necessary equipment and trained
    personnel -- if not already at the clinic -- should be sent to the
    clinic in order to stabilize enough for transfer to a higher
    medical facility.

C. Once the rewarming process has started in the clinic, it should
    be continued with slow, gradual techniques until transfer is
    possible and appropriate.

HYPOTHERMIA: HOSPITAL

A. Some General Points

   1. Treat to the level of your ability as your hospital equipment, staff and skills dictate.

   2. All patients should be stabilized before any transport to another facility. The patient should be kept in the sending hospital until the patient is stable.

B. Evaluation

   1. Initial attention to the ABCs and CPR as needed.

   2. Vital signs, including rectal temperature.

   3. Brief history.

   4. Brief physical exam:
       a. Feel for skin coldness or warmth.
       b. Level of consciousness.
       c. Cardiopulmonary exam.
       d. Associated trauma.

   5. Suggested laboratory and x-ray evaluation, depending on available staffing and equipment:
       a. Chest x-ray.
       b. 12 lead electrocardiogram.
       c. Urine: urinalysis, sodium and osmolality.
       d. Blood: CBC, BUN, creatinine, electrolytes, sugar, platelets, PTT, prothrombin tine, liver function tests, amylase.
       e. Arterial blood gases.
       f. Weight.

C.   Monitoring and Treatment

    1.   Basic treatment is the same as indicated for prehospital personnel in these guidelines.

    2.   Cardiopulmonary monitoring.

    3.   An I.V. and/or central venous pressure line (in the superior vena cava, not the right heart), with D_5W at 75 cc's per hour. I.V. fluid and rate of infusion will vary depending on the patient's level of hydration and laboratory data.

    4.   Urinary bladder catheter.

    5.   Nasogastric tube, if the patient is unconscious and the airway is protected.

    6.   Endotracheal/Nasotracheal tube is indicated in the unconscious patient after careful neck evaluation.

    7.   Daily weights: I & O.

    8.   Always ventilate with warm, moist air or oxygen. (Typical unwarmed ventilation is approximately 72 degrees F. [22 degrees C.].)

    9.   Sodium bicarbonate administration is based on arterial blood gases.

   10.   Continue monitoring until stable and warm.

D. Adding Heat

1. The recommendation possibilities include:

External Methods	Internal Methods

a. Gradual spontaneous a. Warm steam inhalation/
    rewarming.   ventilation.
b. Warming blankets,   b. Peritoneal lavage.
    warming mattresses,   c. Warm I.V. fluids.
    etc.   d. Extracorporeal
c. Tub bath.   circulation (AV shunt).

2. Regardless of the method chosen for adding heat, the patient must be under total physiologic control, to allow you to deal with the metabolic needs of the patient.

3. Tub bath is one of the most rapid methods and requires immediate laboratory results and extremely close physiological monitoring to maintain control of the situation.

4. Do not compromise extremity circulation by using tourniquets, pneumatic antishock garments or ice packs.

    Note: Pneumatic antishock garments are not indicated for hypothermia, but may be used to treat hypovolemic shock in a hypothermic patient.

5. The recommended temperature is about 105 to 110 degrees F. (40 to 43 degrees C.) for all methods.

6. For Severe Hypothermia without Signs of Life (Requiring CPR)

    Warm the core as rapidly as you can handle, using one or more of the methods. (For example, warming mattress, warm steam inhalation, and peritoneal lavage), trying to get the patient warmer than approximately 85 degrees F. (30 degrees C.).

7. For Severe Hypothermia with Life Signs

    Use your judgment, utilizing one or more of the methods.

E.   Most Common Problems

Note: Drug therapy should be moderated because in the cold patient medications are both inefficient and poorly metabolized.

1.   Arrhythmias — these are usually atrial arrhythmias:

a.   If patient is very cold, these atrial arrhythmias will usually convert spontaneously with rewarming.

b.   If the temperature is rising and the arrhythmia does not convert, you may want to use the usual antiarrhythmic medication.

c.   If the treatment is not working, add more heat.

d.   Ventricular fibrillation in the very cold patient is treated with CPR, adding heat, and cardioversion after the temperature reaches approximately 85 degrees F. (30 degrees C.).

e.   In the patient whose temperature is rising, the standard treatment for ventricular fibrillation should be utilized (AHA, others).

2.   Dehydration: Monitor and treat accordingly.

3.   Hyperkalemia: Monitor and treat accordingly. (Do not infuse potassium in I.V.'s.)

4.   Hyperglycemia: Monitor and treat accordingly.

F.   Transferring Patients to Tertiary Care Facilities

  1.   The general indications to transfer the patient from a smaller hospital to a tertiary care facility are:

        a.   Lack of nursing and support staff.
        b.   Lack of equipment to properly provide for a critically ill patient.

  2.   Specifically, the patient should be transferred if:

        a.   There is no capability for rapid arterial blood gas results.
        b.   There is profound neurological depression.
        c.   There is associated significant trauma.

  3.   The patient should not be transferred until stable.

COLD WATER NEAR DROWNING:
GENERAL POINTS

A.   Anyone submerged long enough to be unconscious and/or require CPR, who has been under water less than one hour, should be sent to the hospital.

B.   If the person has been under water for more than one hour, no attempt at resuscitation should be made.

C.   If it is not known how long the person has been under water, we should consider them to have been under water less than one hour.

D.   There is no difference between fresh and salt water near drowning regarding outcome or treatment.

E.   These principles apply to any near drowning, not just those in cold water. The difference between warm and cold water is that in submersions greater than 6 minutes, the chance for survival in warm water is much less than in cold water. The colder the water, the better the chance for survival.

F.   Because the level of coldness is rarely profound (below 85 degrees F. / 30 degrees C.) in cold water near drowning, the hypothermia aspect of the problem is less critical than the pulmonary or coagulation aspects. Thus, rewarming is done very cautiously and gradually, without the need for invasive techniques such as peritoneal lavage or AV shunts.

G.   Many near drowning victims die of a particular type of disseminated intravascular coagulation, not from their pulmonary problems.

COLD WATER NEAR DROWNING:
FIRST RESPONDER/GENERAL PUBLIC

Evaluation and Treatment

1. It is very important to clear the airway with any of the standard maneuvers, but no specific maneuvers are mandatory to expel water from the lungs. Do not do the Heimlich maneuver on these patients.

2. CPR must be started immediately.

3. Assess carefully for associated injuries.

4. Follow the first responder section on Hypothermia (except for the two minute pulse check) for additional therapy as needed (See page 119.)

COLD WATER NEAR DROWNING: EMERGENCY MEDICAL TECHNICIAN I

Evaluation and Treatment

1. It is very important to clear the airway with any of the standard maneuvers, but no specific maneuvers are mandatory to expel water from the lungs. Do not do the Heimlich maneuver on these patients.

2. CPR must be started immediately.

3. Assess carefully for associated injuries.

4. Follow the Emergency Medical Technician I section on Hypothermia (except for the two minute pulse check) for additional therapy as needed. (See page 123.)

COLD WATER NEAR DROWNING:
EMERGENCY MEDICAL TECHNICIAN II

Evaluation and Treatment

1. It is very important to clear the airway with any of the standard maneuvers, but no specific maneuvers are mandatory to expel water from the lungs. Do not do the Heimlich maneuver on these patients.

2. CPR <u>must</u> be started immediately.

3. Assess carefully for associated injuries.

4. Follow the Emergency Medical Technician II section on Hypothermia (except for the two minute pulse check) for additional therapy as needed. (See page 127.)

COLD WATER NEAR DROWNING: EMERGENCY MEDICAL TECHNICIAN III

Evaluation and Treatment

1. It is very important to clear the airway with any of the standard maneuvers, but no specific maneuvers are mandatory to expel water from the lungs. Do not do the Heimlich maneuver on these patients.

2. CPR must be started immediately.

3. Assess carefully for associated injuries.

4. Follow the Emergency Medical Technician III section on Hypothermia (except for the two minute pulse check) for additional therapy as needed. (See page 132.)

COLD WATER NEAR DROWNING: PARAMEDIC

Evaluation and Treatment

1. It is very important to clear the airway with any of the standard maneuvers, but no specific maneuvers are mandatory to expel water from the lungs. Do not do the Heimlich maneuver on these patients.

2. CPR must be started immediately.

3. Assess carefully for associated injuries.

4. Follow the Paramedic section on Hypothermia (except for the two minute pulse check) for additional therapy as needed. (See page 137.)

COLD WATER NEAR DROWNING: SMALL/BUSH CLINIC

Evaluation and Treatment

1. It is very important to clear the airway with any of the standard maneuvers, but no specific maneuvers are mandatory to expel water from the lungs. Do not do the Heimlich maneuver on these patients.

2. CPR must be started immediately.

3. Assess carefully for associated injuries.

4. Follow the Small/Bush Clinics section on Hypothermia for additional therapy as needed. (See page 142.)

COLD WATER NEAR DROWNING: HOSPITAL

A. Evaluation

The evaluation is generally the same as indicated in the Hypothermia: Hospital section (see page 143) except for the laboratory evaluation, which in near drowning should be, in order:

1. Arterial blood gases.
2. Chest x-ray.
3. 12 lead electrocardiogram.
4. Electrolytes, BUN, CBC.
5. Scan the serum for pinkness (indicating hemolysis).
6. Institute cardiorespiratory monitoring.
7. I.V. therapy - D_5W at keep open levels. (In children, 1/4 - 1/2 maintenance rate.)

B.   Therapy

1.   Attention to the ABC's, with respiratory support, intubation, etc., as needed.

2.   Rewarming. Active rewarming methods (warm air inhalation, external heat sources, etc.) should be used only while CPR is required.

Once circulation has been established, do only passive rewarming (light sheets or light blankets; room temperature). Note that these patients often become hyperthermic.

3.   Aspiration pneumonitis and pulmonary edema may be treated with:

a.   Corticosteroids.
b.   Penicillin.
c.   Lasix.

4.   Profound neurological depression: Recommend cerebral resuscitation, as per Conn*, with intraventricular pressure monitoring, diuretics and barbiturates.

5.   Hemolysis — Treat as with any patient with hemolysis.

6.   Disseminated Intravascular Coagulation — Treat as with any patient with DIC.

7.   Renal insufficiency — Treat as with any patient with renal insufficiency.

* "Cerebral Salvage in Near Drowning following Neurological Classification by Triage," A.W. Conn, Canadian Anesthesia Society Journal, Volume 27, No. 3, May, 1980.

C.   Transferring the Near Drowning Patient to Tertiary Care
     Facility

     1.   First the patient should be stabilized at the nearest hospital
          with intubation as necessary, and ventilation.

     2.   The general indications to transfer the patient from a small
          hospital to a tertiary care facility are:

          a.   Lack of nursing and support staff.
          b.   Lack of equipment to properly provide ongoing care
               for a critically ill patient.

     3.   Specifically, the patient should be transferred if:

          a.   There is no capability for rapid arterial blood gas
               results.
          b.   There is deterioration of pulmonary status.
          c.   There is renal insufficiency.
          d.   There is hemolysis.
          e.   There is profound neurological depression.
          f.   There is associated significant trauma.

     4.   Air transport should be in an aircraft pressurized to sea
          level or flying at sea level. You may need to increase
          oxygen supplementation depending on the level of pres-
          surization.

COLD WATER NEAR DROWNING: HOSPITAL

Appendix II

INSULATION — THE "CLO UNIT"

The clo is formally defined by the following equation:

$$I = [c(T_h-T_c) (A) (t)]/H$$

Where:

I = Thermal resistance

T_h = The temperature of the hot side

T_c = The temperature of the cold side

A = the area

H = The heat transferred

t = The time

c = A proportionality constant to adjust the units to those desired.

If T_h and T_c are in °C, A in m^2, H in Kcal, then c = 5.55 and I is in clo.

If T_h and T_c are in °F, A in ft^2, t in hrs., H in BTU, then c = 1.136 I is still in clo. This also defines the conversion factor from the engineers "R" value to the clo.

The above formal definition of the clo was originally derived by A.P. Gagge, et al*, from consideration of human comfort and clothing requirements. They assumed that a normal, average human seated quietly in a 21°C (70°F) room would be comfortable if he were in thermal equilibrium with his surroundings and would be wearing 1 clo of clothing. Knowing the surface area of the average man (1.8m^2), the metabolism rate (50 Kcal/hr m^2), the skin temperature (32°C) and that 76% of the heat loss occurs through the clothing, it was possible to calculate the total thermal resistance. From other experiments it was known that with little air movement the still air layer next to the skin has a thermal resistance of about (.14°C) (hr) (m^2)/Kcal. Subtracting this from the measured value of .324°C hr. m^2/Kcal leaves a thermal resistance of .18°C hr. m^2/Kcal for the clo of clothing the person was assumed to be wearing.

* Gagge, A.P. Barton A.C., and Bazett, H.C.: Science 94:428, 1941

Conversion factors for thermal resistance and transmission units

RESISTANCE UNITS

FROM	MULTIPLY BY	TO GET
$L\,I_{clo}$	.648	r_c (°C sec. m^2)/Kcal
I_{clo}	.88	R (°F hr. ft^2)/BTU
I_{clo}	.18	r_m (°C hr. m^2)/Kcal
r_m (°C hr. m^2)/Kcal	5.56	I_{clo}
R (°F hr. ft^2)/BTU	1.136	I_{clo}

TRANSMISSION UNITS

FROM	DO	TO GET
I_{clo}	$1.54/I_{clo}$	t_c Kcal/(°C sec. m^2)
I_{clo}	$1.136/I_{clo}$	U BTU/(°F hr. ft^2)
I_{clo}	$5.56/I_{clo}$	t_m Kcal/(°C hr. m^2)
I_{clo}	$6.45/I_{clo}$	t_w watt/°C m^2
U BTU/(°F hr. ft^2)	1.136/U	I_{clo}
T t_w watt/ (°C m^2)	$6.45/t_w$	I_{clo}
t_m Kcal/ (°C hr. m^2)	$6.56/t_m$	I_{clo}
t_c Kcal/ (°C sec. m^2)	$1.54\,t_c$	I_{clo}

Courtesy 3M Corporation; Edward R. Hauser

GLOSSARY

ACUTE HYPOTHERMIA

Hypothermia of quick onset, generally 6 hours or less. Some authorities feel that 2 hours or less should be classified as "acute" while the period 2 to 6 hours should be called "prolonged" or "sub-acute" hypothermia.

AFTERDROP

The further lowering of the core temperature after the reheating process has begun.

AMBIENT TEMPERATURE

The temperature of the environment - the so called "outside temperature."

ARRHYTHMIA

Irregular rhythm, such as heart rate.

ASYSTOLE

A heart that has stopped, without beating.

ATAXIA

Loss of coordination.

BASAL METABOLIC RATE

The amount of energy required by the resting body to maintain normal physiologic functions.

CALORIE

The amount of heat necessary to raise 1 gram of water 1°C at 15°C.

CEREBELLUM

The portion of the brain that controls balance, coordination, among other reflexes.

CHILBLAIN

An irritated reaction of dry skin to mild cold, discussed in the text.

CHIMETLON

Another term for "chilblain."

CIRCADIAN

The same as diurnal, changing on a 24 hour cycle.

CLO
>A measurement of clothing insulation, discussed in the text and in Appendix II.

COLD DIURESIS
>The loss of body fluid through urination when cold stressed. The mechanism is discussed in the text.

CONDUCTION
>The direct transfer of heat from one object to another.

CONVECTION
>The transfer of heat by the movement of a liquid or gas.

CORE
>The vital interior of the body consisting of the organs, most notably the heart, lungs, and brain.

COUNTERCURRENT HEAT EXCHANGE
>A method of heat preservation whereby returning venous blood is directed to a deeper set of veins that run along side arteries. Heat from the artery helps increase the temperature of the returning blood, while the arterial blood cools on its outward journey.

CPR
>Cardio-pulmonary resuscitation. Its uses in hypothermia are discussed in the text.

CRYSTALLIZATION, LATENT HEAT OF
>See "fusion, latent heat of."

DIURNAL
>Changing daily. Many body functions have a diurnal change. The resting temperature is one of them.

DROWNING
>Death by suffocation under water.

DROWNPROOFING
>A technique of remaining afloat without a life jacket, discussed in the text.

ENDOGENOUS
>Controlled or originating from within.

EQUIVALENT CHILL TEMPERATURE
>An expression in degrees of temperature which represents the feeling of cold due to the effect of wind currents.

EVAPORATION
Changing from a liquid to a gas.

EVAPORATION, LATENT HEAT OF
The amount of heat required to change a liquid to a gas without an increase in the temperature of the substance. To evaporate water it requires 540 kcal per liter (2.2 pounds).

FIBRILLATION
Quivering. In heart muscle an arrhythmia that produces a very erratic heart rate, if it is atrial; or a pre-lethal heart rhythm which allows no effective blood movement, if it is ventricular.

FROST NIP
Superficial surface freezing of tissue.

FROSTBITE
The freezing of tissue, discussed in the text.

FROZEN LUNG
Not a freezing process of the lung, but a pulmonary irritation caused by very cold air, discussed in the text

FUSION, LATENT HEAT OF
The amount of heat required to melt a solid to a liquid state, such as snow to water, without raising the temperature of the substance. This equals 79.7 kcal per kilogram (2.2 pounds) of ice.

H.E.L.P.
Heat escape lessening posture, a method of heat preservation when immersed alone in cold water. Discussed in the text.

HOMEOTHERM
An organism, such as a mammal, which must maintain its internal body temperature within a narrow range. For humans this is 96° to 101°F (35.5° to 38°C).

HUDDLE
A method of heat preservation when immersed with a group in cold water, discussed in the text.

HUNTING RESPONSE
A popular term for "cold induced vasodilation," the sporadic opening of constricted blood vessels. Described in the text.

HYPOTHALAMUS
A portion of the brain that controls temperature regulation among other regulatory functions.

HYPOTHERMIA
   The lowering of the body temperature to 95°F (35°C) or lower.

IMMERSION
   In water up to the head.

IMMERSION FOOT
   Trench foot, a wet cold injury of the foot. Discussed in the text.

IMMERSION HYPOTHERMIA
   Hypothermia from immersion in cold water. As it is very quick in onset, it is a form of acute hypothermia.

INUIT
   The proper name for "eskimo," and used throughout this text. The Inuit consider the term "eskimo" derogatory.

KILOCALORIE
   One thousand calories. A unit of metabolic measurement, the so called "calorie" referred to in diets.

KIBE
   A form of chilblain with cracking of the skin.

KCAL
   Kilocalorie.

MAMMALIAN DIVING REFLEX
   A method of heat and oxygen conservation found in many diving mammals and some youngsters. Discussed in the text.

MANTLE
   The outer surface layers of the body. The outer mantle consists of skin and subcutaneous fat. The inner mantle consists of muscle. As opposed to the body "core."

METABOLIC ICEBOX
   A term for describing the relatively stable condition of the profoundly hypothermic individual.

MICRO-ENVIRONMENT
   The area immediately surrounding an object.

NEAR DROWNING
   Survival for at least 24 hours after a drowning episode.

PERNIO
   Another term for "chilblain."

POIKILOTHERM
An animal which varies its temperature according to the surrounding temperature, the so called cold blooded animals and plants.

POSTMORTEM
After death, at autopsy.

RADIATION
Heat transfer by the emission of infra-red energy.

SPECIFIC DYNAMIC ACTION OF FOOD
The energy used in the metabolic processing and digestion of food.

SUBMERSION
In water over the head.

SUBMERSION HYPOTHERMIA
Hypothermia from submersion in cold water. As it is very quick in onset, it is a form of acute hypothermia. As the victim is under water, it will result in near drowning or drowning.

THERMOGENESIS
The formation of heat.

THERMOREGULATION
The control of temperature.

TRENCH FOOT
See the text under "immersion foot."

VAPOR BARRIER
A technique of preventing the skin from breathing and transmitting moisture to clothing or the outside atmosphere.

VAPORIZATION, LATENT HEAT OF
The same as "latent heat of evaporation."

VASOCONSTRICTION
The clamping down or narrowing of blood vessels.

VASODILATATION
An alternate spelling for "vasodilation."

VASODILATION
The opening of blood vessels to maximum diameter.

VOLITIONAL WORK
Work performed by desire to accomplish a task. Purposeful exercise.

WIND CHILL FACTOR
The amount of heat lost due to convection by wind currents at specific ambient temperatures. This complex subject is covered in the text.

SUGGESTED READING

Over 200 articles, many lecture and seminar notes, many personal conversations have been synthesized into this book. The following I regard as amongst the most informative. They in turn have extensive biographical lists that differ according to the particular interests of the author.

AUERBACH, PAUL S., and EDWARD C. GEEHR, *Management of Wilderness and Environmental Emergencies*, Macmillan Publishing Company, New York, 1983.

BANGS, CAMERON, "Disturbances Due to Cold," *Current Therapy* by Conn, ed., pages 910-918, WB Saunders Company, Philadelphia, 1980. *Review the entire series of books published by Saunders under the title "Current Therapy." A different author is responsible for this section yearly.*

BANGS, CAMERON and MURRAY HAMLET, "Out in the Cold - Management of Hypothermia, Immersion, and Frostbite," *Topics in Emergency Medicine*, Aspen Systems Corporation, pages 19-37, 1980.

KREIDER, MARLIN, "Hypothermia: Latest Findings, Newest Treatments," *Appalachia* Vol XLIII No 2, pages 18-39, Dec 1980.

LATHROP, THEODORE, *Hypothermia: Killer of the Unprepared*, Mazamas, Portland, Oregon, 1975.

POZOS, ROBERT S., and DAVID O. BORN, *Hypothermia*, New Century Publishers, Inc., Piscataway, NJ, 1982.

POZOS, ROBERT S. and LORENTZ W. WITTMERS, JR., Editors, *The Nature and Treatment of Hypothermia*, University of Minnesota Press, Minneapolis, 1983.

REULER, JAMES B., "Hypothermia: Pathophysiology, Clinical Settings, and Management," *Annals of Internal Medicine*, Vol 89, pages 519-527, 1978.

ROLNICK, MICHAEL, et al "Frostbite," *Consultant*, pages 133-139, Dec 1980.

WASHBURN, BRADFORD, *Frostbite*, Museum of Science, Boston, 1963.

WELTON, DAVID E., et al, "Treatment of Profound Hypothermia," *Journal American Medical Association*, Vol 240, No 21, page 2291, Nov 1978.

Extensive use was made of the Technical Bulletins of the 3M Corporation, Minneapolis, Minnesota, with regard to the mathematics of the "Clo" equation, thermography results of clothing construction, and certain aspects of synthetic fiber properties. Additional fabric and fiber technical data was obtained from various manufacturers. Certain individual references are listed when appropriate in the text.

INDEX

Books available through Indiana Camp Supply, Inc., P.O. Box 344, Pittsboro, Indiana 46167. Check, money order, VISA, Mastercard and American Express accepted; please include expiration date of card. Write or call (317) 892-3307.

Commercial orders must be addressed to Stackpole Books, P.O. Box 1831, Cameron and Kelker Streets, Harrisburg, Pennsylvania 17105. For fast service use the toll free number. Call 1-800-READ NOW. For library telemarketing orders, call 1-800-LIBRARI. In Pennsylvania, call (717) 234-5041. Please call between 8:30 a.m. and 4:00 p.m. EST.

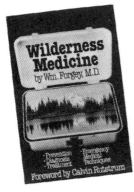

WILDERNESS MEDICINE
William W. Forgey, M.D.

An informative medical procedures manual written specifically for outdoorsmen interested in preventing, diagnosing and treating common illnesses and injuries. Emergency medical and surgical techniques are described in simple terms. Devoted to the selection of medications, both prescription and non-prescription and their use under wilderness conditions. **Paperback**, 5½ x 8½, 120 pages, photos, diagrams, illus. 0-934802-14-9 **$9.95** Canadian $12.95

"... a clear, concise guide to treating the gamut of outdoor mishaps, from insect bites and fishhook removal to more serious problems such as broken bones and heatstroke."
Sports Afield 11/84

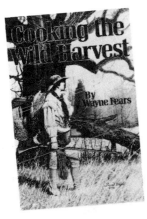

COOKING THE WILD HARVEST
J. Wayne Fears

Over 250 recipes recommended by various agricultural universities' Cooperative Extension Service home economists. Fears combines his talents as a wildlife biologist, outdoorsman, and prize-winning outdoor writer for hints on proper field dressing and procuring. **Paperback**, 6x9, 185 pages. 0-934802-14-9 **$12.95** Canadian $15.95

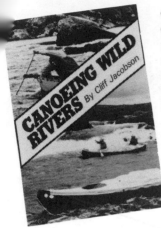

CANOEING WILD RIVERS
Cliff Jacobson
An easy reading manual, of source material, canoeing tips, advanced techniques, and gear recommendations by a weathered expert. **Paperback**, 340 pages, color photos, illus.
0-934802-17-3 **$14.95** Canadian 17.95

> "If you've ever dreamed of canoeing Alaska's arctic rivers, or for that matter, any waterway in North America, then **Canoeing Wild Rivers** is the first book you should obtain."
> Alaska Outoors 11/84

> "This book, **Canoeing Wild Rivers,** by Cliff Jacobson is the one I recommend above all others ... It is not a re-hash of previous writers, but the accumulated learnings of much personal experience."
> Verlen Kruger ['84]
> Ultimate Canoe Challenge member

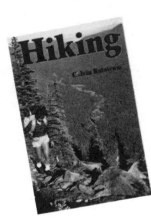

HIKING
Calvin Rutstrum
A comprehensive, procedural coverage from the short urban walk to the extensive wilderness trek, with analysis of equipment, outdoor living methods, and modern hiking ethics. **Paperback**, 6x9, 125 pages, photos, illus.
0-934802-20-3 **$8.95** Canadian $11.95

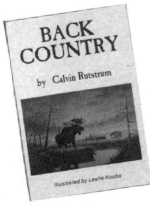

BACK COUNTRY
Calvin Rutstrum
A volume of adventures, trips and events from the Northern Wilderness during the first part of this century. **Paperback**, 6x9, 255 pages, Les Kouba illus.
0-934802-11-4 **$14.95** Canadian $17.95

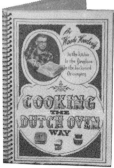

COOKING THE DUTCH OVEN WAY
Woody Woodruff
Written by a designer/manufacturer of dutch ovens, and a 50-year Scouter and life-long camper and hiker. Recipes for good old fashioned dishes and baker's favorites, easily prepared at home or in the north-woods. **Paperback**, 6x9, 142 pages, illus.
0-934802-01-7 **$8.95** Canadian $11.95

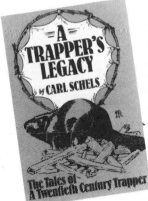

A TRAPPER'S LEGACY
Carl Schels
A rare glimpse of a professional trapper's life, difficulties, and dangers of existence deep in the wilderness. Forced into poverty by the Great Depression, Carl Schels decided to chase his dream of wilderness living and survived to write this story -- his legacy. **Paperback**, 5½ x 8½, 212 pages, photos.
0-934802-12-2 **$9.95** Canadian $12.95

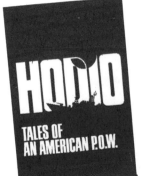

HODIO
C.N. Day
The true story of a 19-year-old American seaman captured off the shores of Burma during a naval battle of World War II. For the 42 months in brutal prison camps of Indonesia, **HODIO** became synonymous with Prisoner of War. **Paperback**, 5½ x 8½, 216 pages.
0-934802-13-0 **$9.95** Canadian $12.95

DATE DUE

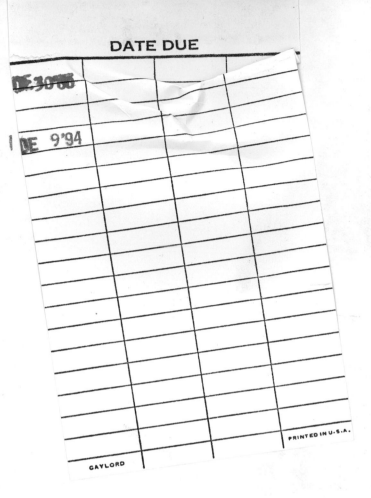

DE 3U88			
DE 9'94			
			PRINTED IN U.S.A.

GAYLORD

AAS 8972